PROFESSIONALS AND PARENTS

Managing Children's Behaviour

CHARLES GIBB AND
PETER RANDALL

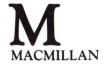

MACMILLAN

First published 1989

Published by
MACMILLAN EDUCATION LTD
Houndmills, Basingstoke, Hampshire RG21 2XS
and London
Companies and representatives
throughout the world

Typeset by Footnote Graphics,
Warminster, Wilts
Printed in Hong Kong

British Library Cataloguing in Publication Data
Gibb, Charles
Professionals and parents
1. Children. Behavioural disorders
I. Title   II. Randall, Peter
618.92'89
ISBN 0–333–48996–9
pack of Handout pages ISBN 0–333–49458–X

M

£8·95

Professionals and parents

About the authors

Charles Gibb and Peter Randall are educational psychologists. Charles Gibb read psychology at the University of Dundee, graduating with an MA, and educational psychology at the University of Edinburgh, graduating with an MSc. He gained a DipEd at what is now the Northern College in Aberdeen. Peter Randall has a BSc in psychology from the University of Hull, and an MSc in educational psychology from the University of Manchester. They are members of the British Psychological Society. Both have a special interest in pre-school children and have worked extensively in this field with parents and with other professionals for whom they have run courses on the behaviour and development of young children. They have published many articles in the professional and academic journals, jointly and individually. In addition, Peter Randall is an honorary staff member of the Department of Social Policy and Professional Studies of the University of Hull and is the author of *Infant Screening: A Handbook For Teachers* also published by Macmillan.

Contents

Introduction

Who is this intended for?

The course is designed for any professional group who may be asked by parents for advice and help in managing infant behaviour problems at home and for residential professionals who care for infants.

Health visitors
Field social workers
Nursery nurses
Playgroup organisers
Students in training
School nurses
Residential social workers
Child guidance workers
Educational welfare officers
Educational psychologists
Nursery teachers

The course is also designed to be used with parents in, for example, 'parenting skills' groups.

What age group of children is covered?

The course is concerned with infants aged up to five years.
This is the time at which children learn most about the standards of behaviour in our society. We continue to learn throughout life, of course, but the years up to the age of five are the richest.

What is the overall aim?

The overall aim is to establish a practical knowledge of management methods for use with young children who present behaviour or management problems, and to provide training in how these methods can be transmitted to the primary managers—parents.

What does the course contain?

The course contains five parts, ordered chronologically. The first four parts represent the goals of the course. Each goal is subserved by a set of smaller-step objectives. The fifth part provides an opportunity to put these to the test. The content of the parts in terms of goals and objectives is as follows.

PART 1   *Goal*

To define the need for a structured, systematic approach to infant management problems.

Objectives

1   To teach problem definition skills.
2   To introduce the idea of behaviour problems as faulty learning.
3   To teach effective analysis of behaviour problems.

Multiple choice test on Part 1.

PART 2   *Goal*

To teach suitable methods of intervention with the problem behaviours of young children.

Objectives

1   To teach the use of contingent reinforcers and punishers.
2   To teach a set of specific techniques.
3   To introduce some methods of recording behaviour.

Multiple choice test on Part 2.

PART 3   *Goal*

To provide an organised framework for intervention with families.

Objectives

1   To teach a list of ten steps to setting up a programme of intervention.
2   To provide an example of the ten steps in a real-life situation.

Multiple choice test on Part 3.

PART 4   *Goal*

To provide a method of parent training.

Objectives

1   To stress the role of parents in bringing about change.
2   To provide a protocol for transmission of problem management skills to parents.
3   To highlight boobytraps and pitfalls in parent training.

Multiple choice test on Part 4.

PART 5   An exercise based on the material in the first four parts.

Key features of the course material

The top outside corner of every working page is labelled to remind instructors and other readers of exactly where they are in the course as they work through it.

Pages headed Handout are intended primarily for use when the course is being completed by groups of students under the guidance of an instructor or course leader. However, they are an integral part of the course and as such are also for use by individual readers. Handout pages are also available as single sheets in a shrink-wrapped pack (ISBN 0–333–49458–X).

All other working pages are text pages which contain material that reinforces and expands on the handouts. Text pages represent the teaching content.

Instructor boxes are distributed at strategic intervals throughout the manual. They are for use by instructors when the course is being used with groups of trainees and explain how to make use of particular text pages and handouts. Every part of the manual is covered by a number of instructor boxes.

How is the course used?

As an instructor of groups

Instructors should read through all the material before using it with students/trainees in order to get a general idea of thinking and direction, and to familiarise themselves with the layout and organisation. They should also gather together all the materials necessary to teach the course (eg overhead projector equipment, sufficient handouts and so on). They may also want to gather together other material to suit their own modifications and preferences, if any (eg blackboard and copies of their own examples). This last point is important since it will be seen from reading through the course that for those who wish it, there is considerable flexibility of approach. This is to ensure that instructors can modify while retaining the general path.

This settled, it is then for instructors to use the **text** both to guide the trainees through the **handouts**, and as source material for lecturing or workshops. In both these inseparable activities, more specific guidelines are provided in the **instructor boxes**.

It is expected that instructors will become increasingly familiar with the material as they teach to more groups. This means the need to refer to the text and instructor boxes will diminish over time.

One of the important considerations for instructors will be timescale. For completion of this course there are no hard and fast rules on timing. We have completed the first four parts in one day with groups of experienced trainees, though this makes for a very hard and long day. We have also used a more leisurely 3-month period for trainees at the beginning of their professional careers. Instructors should select a time-scale to suit their own needs and those of their students. However, it is vital to be thoroughly familiar with the whole course content and requirements before deciding on a time-scale.

As an individual reader

This is simply a matter of reading the material through from start to finish—as if it were a book—and completing all the exercises on the way. The individual reader should, however, omit the instructor boxes since these may introduce confusion and possible solutions to problems before they occur in the text.

The individual reader who, in the absence of an instructor, wishes to find out more about these issues and practices may find the further reading sections at the end of each part particularly useful.

PART 1

> **To define the need for a structured, systematic approach to infant management problems**

This goal is subserved by three objectives:

1 To teach problem definition skills.
2 To introduce the idea of behaviour problems as a consequence of faulty learning.
3 To teach the effective analysis of behaviour problems

These are followed by a multiple choice questionnaire on Part 1.

Objective 1

To teach problem definition skills

It is often the case that parents experiencing management difficulties present their request for help along with a welter of problems, anxieties, complaints and sometimes mis-information that they think the listener wants to hear. It is vital that you 'refine' all this melée of fact and fiction to an exact definition of the problem or problems. How else will you know what you are trying to change and whether you can help or not?

The material relating to Objective 1 is designed to assist with problem definition.

INSTRUCTOR 1

If you are running a group training workshop you may ask your trainees to read the passage in Handout 1 and augment the information by asking you any questions they like. You can take the part of anyone in the family or involved in it (eg father, mother, family doctor etc). Feel free to make up answers, perhaps using a family situation you are familiar with. Your 'made-up' answers must not contradict information in the passage, or help the trainees answer the questions which follow. When they have finished ask them to answer the five questions. It is important to emphasise brevity and to allow no more than 20 minutes. Give further explanations if necessary.

═══ HANDOUT 1 ═══

The Smith family

The following case history of a family with many problems is expressed in the words of a social services case conference report. Inevitably you will have questions that the material does not answer. Given this difficulty, use your experience to fill in these gaps as best you can. When you have read all the information carefully, answer the questions at the end.

1   The family consists of:

Mr George Smith, 36 years old, unemployed for 2½ years

Mrs Susan Smith, 25 years old, housewife

Amy Smith, 11 months old

Keith Smith, 4 years old

Andrew Smith, 15 years old, currently in the closed unit of a community home with education.

2   Mr Smith has been married twice and Andrew is his son by his first marriage. It ended in a stormy divorce after three years when the first Mrs Smith walked out, leaving the then 4-year-old Andrew locked in a wardrobe. She has had no real contact since but occasionally rings up Mr Smith and Andrew to enquire how her 'bairn' is getting on. She sounds intoxicated and frequently weeps. These telephone calls provoke long and furious rows between Mr Smith and his second wife.

Mr Smith is unemployed. He says he was made redundant from his storeman job but Mrs Smith says he was sacked for being drunk. He seems to spend most of his day doing little other than occasionally walking to the pub (usually in the middle of a row) where he can spend up to 3 hours. He has had only sporadic, unskilled labour work since leaving school but he did have, for 18 months, a job as a taxi driver with a friend. He claims this was the best time of his life.

He seems to be a bit strange and possibly mildly depressed.

Mr Smith complains that Mrs Smith is frigid. They have little or no sexual contact and only rarely do they express their feelings for each other.

He is begging for help. His financial state is bad and poor management has led to lump sum payments from the DHSS to cover electricity and other bills. He is terrified that Keith is 'going the same way as Andrew' and feels frustrated and emasculated, because he cannot control either of his sons' behaviour.

3   Mrs Susan Smith is considerably younger. She had had many boyfriends before meeting Mr Smith and lived with him for about one year before they married, five months before Keith was born.

Mrs Smith is attractive in a jaded way and exudes a cheerful demeanour that is out of proportion to the magnitude of her problems. She complains bitterly about Mr Smith saying that he is 'a lazy, good-for-nothing drunk' whose first wife 'had the best years of him'. She feels that he does not appreciate her and that he should be grateful to have a good looking young wife. At present she is worried about her stretch marks which have not faded since Amy's birth. These embarrass her when she changes at her adult education course of aerobics. She is also concerned that Amy is not putting on weight and that Keith disregards her. She has stopped Keith from having cold drinking chocolate which he adores because a neighbour said the additives might be making him hyperactive. She would like to talk to her own mother about the children, but there is no contact at the moment because Mr Smith told Susan's mother to 'xxxx off' when he thought she was interfering in the family.

Susan is on the pill but wonders why she bothers when her husband is so sexually inactive.

4 Keith is a good looking but scruffy 4-year-old who goes to nursery unit (attached to a primary school) five mornings a week. The staff there say that he is hyperactive and aggressive. They believe that his hostility is caused by frustration; apparently he will not play very long at any activity and his speech is unclear.

At home Keith is a naughty boy and frequently has breath holding tantrums to which his parents have responded by smacking and shouting at him. On one occasion they locked him in a bedroom and he threw a wooden brick through the window and tore down the curtains. He is clearly a very disturbed and emotionally rejected child because he deliberately urinates on the carpets and bedding, refuses to go to bed or stay in his own bed. His tempers at nighttime disturb Amy and also earn bangs on the wall from the irritated but otherwise kindly, elderly couple next door. Keith will play with Amy but woe betide her if she does not hand him toys, her food etc.

Keith has his good side—he laughs a lot and plays in a limited way with a toy garage, cars and some Lego. He is always pleased to see his nursery teacher but is terrified that she will think he is a naughty boy. He likes watching TV with his father and is keen to talk to the latter about the programmes they see together.

5 Amy is a delightful child and is the reason for frequent visits from the heath visitor. She cries a lot and is not putting on weight. Her play seems to lack imagination and she is manifestly terrified of Keith. He seems to intimidate her and he prefers to eat her food and play with her toys.

Her appearance is as ill-kempt as the rest of the home.

6 Andrew, after prolonged and rather unintelligent delinquency, has been placed in the secure unit of a community house with education. He absconds frequently, returning home to display acting-out tendencies. On occasions he seems wistful and quiet but his attitude is definitely and generally antisocial.

HANDOUT 1

Imagine that you are the professional who sees this family regularly. Mr Smith is begging for help and you are concerned about Amy; you feel that you have something to offer (and you have responsibility for the two pre-school children).

Answer the following questions. Write your answers on a sheet of paper which you can keep. Be *brief* because the answers are needed only to explore general trends at this stage.

Question 1 Having decided to try and help what would be your main aims or goals (list no more than three)?

Question 2 What methods would you use (list no more than three)?

Question 3 Write down at least one unsupportable or subjective statement made about each member of this family of five people. (Such statements are usually opinion not supported by quoted evidence.)

Question 4 What could you measure to show that change was occurring (ie how could you 'measure' something or things to determine whether you were successfully meeting the aims/goals you listed for Question 1?

Question 5 Questions 1 to 4 cover considerations necessary for any type of intervention but they are not arranged in a logical, systematic order. Write down the correct order (eg, if you feel that 4 should come first, write 4 1 2 3).

INSTRUCTOR 2

Some trainees may have difficulties in the following areas:

Question 1: What do you mean by aims or goals?
Explanation: That which you would like to achieve by helping the family—it could be something specific like improving Amy's weight or it could be something more general such as changing attitudes.

Question 3: What do you mean by unsupportable or subjective statements?
Explanation: These are statements that have been made without the provision of supporting evidence; for example, Keith is said to be aggressive but the person writing the information has not said why.

Question 4: What does measure mean here? If the family were getting better you would be able to see it.
Explanation: You should write down specifically the areas in which you could see improvements (or deterioration).

Question 5: General questions can arise here. It is possible only to give prompts such as 'Do you think aims should come before methods when you are working out what to do?'

For the next part you need an overhead projector.

Gather in all the written answers from the trainees. Take one question at a time and go through all the trainees' answers to it. For each question try to discover the answer most commonly given.

This can be achieved by taking one trainee's answer sheet and summarising in broad terms on a separate sheet of paper the answers given. Then go through the rest of the answer sheets and when a trainee's answer matches the summary answer add a tick to your summary sheet. If you come across an answer to a question that doesn't fit the headings you've already got, summarise that answer and write it on the master sheet: thereafter put a tally mark against it every time an answer fits it. Do this for all the questions and answers.

You should end up with a list of answers to each question and these should have tally marks against them. Count up the ticks to discover which were most common. For example, question 1 requires trainees to list three main aims; you should now have the three most common aims given by the trainees. Transfer this information to an overhead projector acetate sheet.

While you are doing this, a co-instructor can be discussing the Smith family issues with the trainees.

Now display the information on the screen.

Using applied behavioural analysis to discuss the answers

There are no simple right or wrong answers to our questions, but in order to meet the first objective (to teach problem definition skills), we must adopt a particular stance or 'model of practice' which enables precise analysis of situations.

The model we have adopted is that of applied behavioural analysis (ABA) which is used by behaviourists to define problems and design interventions.

Thus all the answers are examined from the viewpoint of ABA; the aim is not to state whether they are right or wrong, merely to determine if they meet the criteria of this model of practice.

Essentially, ABA is a way of analysing situations to determine which events (antecedents) generally occur before problem behaviour and which events (consequences) generally occur afterwards. By systematically manipulating either the antecedents or consequences it may be possible to reduce the problem behaviours.

This manipulation is called intervention—we do not use the word 'treatment' because it can be confused with medical treatments. Interventions are psychological in origin rather than medical.

Certain factors are very important to ABA:

1 The problem must be observable, ie it must relate to the presence or absence of a 'piece' of behaviour which can be witnessed by an observer.

2 The problem must be describable:, ie the observers must be able to state exactly what they have witnessed.

3 The problem must be recordable, ie the observer must be able to say how frequently it occurs in order to know that the intervention (manipulation of consequences or antecedents) is having an effect (good or bad).

4 The problem must be remediable. There is no value in identifying a problem—even if it is a real one that matches the criteria given in 1, 2, and 3—if you can do nothing about it. For example, a problem defined as 'This child has Down's Syndrome' is valueless when compared with a problem definition such as 'This child has not learned to use a spoon'.

The emphasis is, therefore, on objectivity. Anything that is not objective does not fit within our ABA model.

In order to examine the answers within the ABA methodology we have provided three items of information for each:

1 ABA criteria for usable answers.

2 Some fairly common answers with comments.

3 Examples of usable answers.

You may therefore read the criteria and see if your answer matches them. Then look through the common answers given in the second item and try and relate your answers to them. The comments that follow are intended to help in learning to identify and reject unusable answers. Finally, read the usable answers.

INSTRUCTOR 3

You must clearly understand all the preceding statements about ABA and behaviourism. Many trainees will think that ABA is nothing more than 'behaviour modification', 'behaviour mod' or 'BM'. In fact these are just shorthand labels for a type of practice that is only part of ABA. You must be well acquainted with the materials of Part 2 in order to answer trainees' questions but be careful not to provide information that goes beyond that given above; try to amplify rather than extend the information.

In relation to Question 1 (which is discussed in the following pages), many trainees find it difficult to discard subjectivity entirely in goal setting and still want to set goals to do with changing 'attitudes', 'relationships', and 'perceptions'. The tendency to keep falling into the subjectivity trap usually brings with it a tendency to confuse goals with methods.

If there is confusion between goals and methods, explain that any one goal may be achieved through several different methods.

QUESTION 1   Having decided to try and help, what would be your main aims or goals (list no more than three).

Criteria

ABA requires that the aims and goals from which intervention is designed should be objectively stated. That is, they should relate to observable problems of behaviour. Moreover the aims or goals should be independent of method.

Common answers

1   Refer the family to . . . (social services, child guidance, child psychiatric service etc).

   Comment. This is not an aim—this is a method; the aim underpinning this response is to get another agency to take on the family. This may be perfectly legitimate but not all problems can be referred away.

2   Refer the parents for marriage guidance counselling.

   Comment. This too is not an aim. The unwritten aim here probably is to improve the state of the marriage in the hope that a more united husband/wife partnership will overcome the other difficulties.

3   Help the parents improve their attitude to each other.

Comment. This is an aim and it appears to be objectively stated. But have you ever seen an attitude? If you had complete access to the human body could you cut one out and examine it? The answer is 'no' to both questions. You can infer an attitude only from the behaviour you see.

For example, a person witnesses the following events in a swimming pool: A tall adolescent boy walks purposefully up behind a small coloured child and pushes him strongly into the pool. The adolescent has passed white children of both sexes and all ages to push in this one coloured child. Inference: the adolescent has racially biased attitudes.

Next, however, the coloured child jumps out of the pool, laughing and shouting, 'Do it again, sneak up on me again'. It is clearly a game he enjoys. Later the adolescent is seen buying crisps and coke for the coloured child in the swimming pool cafe. They are laughing and joking.

Inference: the adolescent does not have racially biased attitudes; in fact he has good positive attitudes.

Clearly we cannot set aims of 'changing attitudes'—these are not objective and neither are they stable.

4   Help Mrs Smith to be more loving with Keith.

Comment. If this could be rephrased objectively it would become a helpful goal within the ABA model. For example, 'After intervention, Mrs Smith will show more praising, cuddling and play behaviour towards Keith'. Most people would agree that these behaviours from a parent indicate 'love' for the child who receives them. This re-phrasing has simply deleted the inference word 'loving' which is, at best, unnecessary and, at worst, misleading.

5   Increase Amy's weight.

Comment. Yes, a usable aim because on an objective and recordable variable. This is a no-nonsense statement which some scales could prove the worth of.

6   Stop Keith urinating on the carpet.

Comment. Yes, a usable aim, certainly objective and recordable.

7   Stop Keith being aggressive.

Comment. Some people would think a black look was aggressive others would not. This aim can be re-phrased to state exactly what behaviour has caused him to be described by the nursery teacher as 'aggressive', for example 'Stop Keith kicking and and hitting other children'.

Usable answers

1   At night Keith will go to his own bed and stay there (so that Mr and Mrs Smith have the opportunity to be husband and wife again).

2   Amy will eat her food and play with her toys without having to give them to Keith.

3   Mr and Mrs Smith will speak more quietly to each other and Mr Smith will spend less money at the pub.

4   Mr and Mrs Smith will clean their home and children on an agreed basis.

Comments on usable answers

(a)   The list is by no means exhaustive. Many more objective aims or goals could be expressed.

(b)   These usable answers refer to observable and recordable behaviours. For example, we could see Keith going to his bed and being in his bed. We could also see Amy playing, and we could count the money Mr Smith saved for both parents to spend on cleaning materials which we could watch them using!

(c)   No subjective comments are included. For example, in answer 4 we did not say 'Mr and Mrs Smith will keep their home nice and clean' for by whose standards would we judge them to have met the goal? Professionals have to be wary of applying their own standards. It is wrong for a relatively well off professional person to do this with clients who may be on the bread-line.

(d)   Methods are not mentioned. The question of how goals are to be met is independent of the statement of the goals themselves.

Now write three goals for this family making sure that (a) they are objective and (b) they are independent of method.

QUESTION 2   What methods would you use (list no more than three).

Criteria

ABA involves the scientific application of one of the most robust theories in psychology. This is learning theory. We have already introduced the concept of the manipulation of antecedents and consequences. The means by which we do this constitutes the tried and tested methods evolved from learning theory. From that viewpoint, the criteria for usable answers are:

(a)   The methods manipulate either the antecedents or consequences of the problem behaviour.

(b)   The methods are applied systematically every time the behaviour occurs or is about to occur.

(c)   The effect of the method can be recorded objectively.

Common answers

1   Counsel Mr and Mrs Smith so that they learn to feel better towards each other.

Comments. (a) The method (counselling) is being confused with an aim (... feel better towards each other).

(b) The link between 'feeling better towards each other' and behaviour is tenuous indeed!

2   Keith needs play therapy to stop his rage by expressing his frustration and bringing it out into the open.

Comments. (a) Does he? Why do we assume that rage, aggression, violence are products of frustration? Why doesn't Keith suck his thumb to vent his frustration instead or do something else? Two assumptions, both subjective, are being made here; first that Keith's rage is caused by frustration and, second, that play therapy will draw it out of him.

(b) This method cannot be successfully recorded. For example, if Keith destroys ten brick towers and stabs six dolls with a plastic sword during his play therapy and subsequently attacks only one child during one day at nursery school, are we to record the number of towers, the number of stabs or the number of attacks? Would he have attacked more children at school if he had destroyed only one tower and stabbed only two dolls?

3   Show Mrs Smith how to feed Amy properly.

Comments. (a) Yes, we have got the beginnings of a good idea here. Showing a better way of feeding Amy could indeed fall within the ABA model of practice. It could represent the manipulation of the antecedents that lead to Keith getting Amy's food.

(b) The effects of this can be objectively measured, ie weigh Amy regularly.

Usable answers

1   Whenever Keith has been good for a day Mr Smith should watch a programme on the television with him.

Comments. (a) This manipulates the consequences of good behaviour.

(b) The first word tells us that it is systematic because 'whenever' means 'every time'.

(c) The answer is less satisfactory from the recording viewpoint—what do we mean by being 'good for a day'? If the parents and professional understand and agree what is meant, then recording is possible.

2   Mr and Mrs Smith should make pleasant sexual contact at night with each other after a day without argument.

Comments. (a) Again there is a pleasant manipulation of consequences but

(b) It would be better if the method statement read 'Mr and Mrs Smith should make pleasant sexual contact at night after any day without argument'.

(c) 'Argument' is not the best specification of that which is to be avoided but, as in the last example, consensus agreement is possible.

3   Keith will be praised by his nursery teacher every time she sees him 'working' (ie, doing what he is supposed to be doing).

Comments. (a) This is a clear manipulation of the consequences of desirable behaviour,

(b) Consistency is implied by the 'every time' comment.

(c) The length of time spent 'working' (ie doing the right thing) is certainly recordable.

4   Mrs Smith should thank Mr Smith every time he gets the children ready in the morning.

Comments. (a) Again, the giving of thanks represents the manipulation of the consequences of of a desirable piece of behaviour.

(b) It is easy to see that it is intended to be consistent.

(c) The desired behaviour is obviously recordable by using something like a diary.

5   For two weeks Amy will be given lunch before Keith returns from nursery school.

Comments. (a) This is an example of manipulaiton of antecedents. If the presence of Amy eating her food is the signal (antecedent) for Keith to take it (problem behaviour) then the change of lunch time arrangements leave Keith without the signal or the food to steal.

(b) Consistency is explicit in the same time scale of two weeks.

(c) Recording the outcome is easy in terms of weighing Amy.

Now write down two more possible methods making sure that they fit into the criteria of (a) manipulating antecedents or consequences, (b) they explicitly show consistency and (c) their effects are measurable.

INSTRUCTOR 4

Some people may think the examples of usable answers too trivial for a family with such great problems. Often the attraction of broader approaches like counselling is that they are thought to be able to tackle many massive problems at the same time. 'Making people more adequate' seems to be a grander aim than some simple management objective. However, from little acorns big trees grow and the step by small step approach is more likely to succeed.

QUESTION 3   Write down at least one unsupportable or subjective statement made about each member of this family of five people.

Criteria

A statement of this sort is generally pivoted about a 'label' given by someone as their subjective interpretation of behaviour they have witnessed. The description given of the family is full of these subjective statements, many of which can act as red herrings. In fact much of the detail in the lengthy description of the Smith family that you have read is of absolutely no value in resolving their problems.

Look at the following examples and compare your answers with them.

Mr Smith, lethargic, bit strange, mildly depressed, feels frustrated and emasculated.

Mrs Smith, exudes a cheerful demeanour.

Keith, hyperactive and aggressive, a naughty boy.

Amy, play lacks imagination, appearance is ill-kempt.

Andrew, seems wistful.

Labelling can be a nightmare for the behavioural analyst because it can divert attention away from the real problems. For example, Keith could be referred to a psychologist because he is . . . 'hyperactive and aggressive' or Andrew's 'wistfulness' might be interpreted by someone else as indicative of a psychiatric problem. These labels have to be deliberately excluded in order to define the problem(s) exactly. Any statement containing such labels is called a 'fuzzy'. Try this little quiz: consider each statement and identify the fuzzies.

1   The problem is that the mother does not relate to her child.

2   The child peels wallpaper from his bedroom wall every morning when he wakes up.

3   The child gives limited eye contact and this had led to a breakdown in the relationship between him and his mother.

4 The problem is that the child throws toys every time he asks for a biscuit and is refused.

5 The problem is that he is jealous of the new baby.

6 The current problem is that the child takes all his clothes off when with his father in the supermarket.

7 Dad gives him a sweet every time he cries.

8 The child is too clingy and insecure.

9 The problem is that he seems not to understand the difference between right and wrong.

10 She pulls her mother's hair whenever she is behind her.

Number 1. You cannot see a mother relating to her child, only the behaviour by which you infer the state of that relationship.

Number 3. What is limited eye contact and how could that directly cause relationship problems?

Number 5. Jealousy is a label here that merely interprets that behaviour.

Number 8. 'Clingy' and 'insecure' are someone's labels for their subjective judgements.

Number 9. Why?

Can you find any other unsupportable statements in the description of the Smith family? Write down at least one.

INSTRUCTOR 5

While this is not conceptually difficult many trainees are reluctant to give up labels that they believe are common sense shorthand. It is important, however, that they realise that one cannot treat labels. In conversation about this family it may be perfectly understandable to say that 'one of Keith's problems is that he is so aggressive' but it is not defining the problem from the viewpoint of intervention. 'Keith hits and kicks any child playing with a toy he wants' is an objective description of the problem and it allows us to decide whether it should take priority over some other problem behaviour.

Attempts to make labels seem urgent by putting qualifiers alongside them (for example, *so* aggressive, *extremely* hyperactive) only disguise the subjectivity of the problem. For example, take two labels attached to another child in a nursery:

1 Paul is extremely aggressive and other parents are complaining that their children come home crying.

2 Paul is hyperactive—we can't keep him at school.

Ostensibly the first of these is the most serious problem but ask the trainees to consider the behaviour actually witnessed by the observer who has applied these labels.

1 Paul shouts angrily and loudly at smaller children who want to play with the toys he is using.

2 Paul regularly runs out of the nursery to play ball in a busy street; he has also run home by himself and was nearly hit by a lorry.

Clearly the problem of the 'aggression' is minor in comparison with the problem of the 'hyperactivity'. Intervention for Paul who, no doubt, has lots of problem behaviours must start with setting his problems in order of importance and that necessitates discarding the subjective labels.

QUESTION 4   What could you measure to show that change was occurring?

Criteria

Anyone who decides to intervene in a family's problems, even though it is at the family's request, has a professional duty to be able to demonstrate the effectiveness (or otherwise) of the methods used. If a doctor treats a patient with high blood pressure he records blood pressure levels before, during and after treatment. ABA requires that these measurements be as objective as possible and taken before, during and after the intervention.

Common answers

1 We could measure improvements in the relationship between Mr and Mrs Smith.

Comments. This is not possible. You cannot see a relationship. You can only see interpersonal behaviour and from it interpret the state of the relationship. Maybe the couple would kiss more frequently or hold hands in the street, or maybe she would make him supper when the children were in bed. Recording such a collection of behaviours, while possible, would prove extremely difficult.

2 We can record the changes in the degree of rejection Mrs Smith shows Keith.

Comment. This is totally dependent upon the ability of the observer to quantify 'degree of rejection'.

3 We can count the number of times Keith wets the carpet.

Comment. Yes. An exact behaviour that can be counted.

4 We can record Amy getting heavier.

Comment. Yes. The child's weight presents the ultimate in scales of measurement.

Usable answers

1   Count the number of nights each week that Keith spends in his own bed.

2   Record the time each day that Keith spends watching television.

3   Record the time that Amy spends playing with her toys when Keith is in the nursery.

4   Count the number of items of family clothing washed each week by one or other parents.

These types of record have all been used at one time or another by the authors. They are all objective and easily obtained.

Please write down two or more objective measurements.

QUESTION 5   Write down question numbers 1–4 in the logical, systematic order necessary to the process of designing an intervention.

Criteria

First we discard all the subjective labels and comments and replace them with objective descriptions of behaviour (3). Next we decide which of these reflect the most pressing problems and which become our aims for intervention (1) and consider how we may record them (4). Finally, we work out our methods for delivering the intervention (2).

INSTRUCTOR 6

If the trainees have come to this point successfully they have mastered the first objective of Goal 1; they now have good problem definition skills. Return to any parts that cause residual difficulties and repeat them before moving to the second objective.

Objective 2

To introduce the idea of behaviour problems as a consequence of faulty learning

'I don't know where he gets it from!' Parents search for causes when their offspring pose serious behaviour problems and get beyond their control. We live in a cause-and-effect world and feel uncomfortable if we cannot discover the reasons for the events that surround us. The need for a reason or cause is even stronger when these events are unpleasant or otherwise undesirable.

Objective 2 is about tackling the myth of internal medical-style causes of bad behaviour.

HANDOUT 2

Thinking about behaviour problems

Traditionally practitioners have considered infant behaviour problems to be symptomatic of underlying disorder—that the problem exists inside the child and must be *diagnosed* and then *treated* with a view to a *cure*. Unfortunately, there is no evidence to suggest that this is anything other than wishful thinking. Even if it were possible to identify a certain causal agent inside someone's head we certainly cannot take off the top of the skull and mend it!

This kind of thinking can lead to curious situations. For example:

1   Infant regularly soils and smears faeces over bedroom wall.

2   Professional *diagnoses cause* as mother's inability to show love to the infant because of her own childhood relationship with her mother.

3   Professional *treats* problem by weekly counselling sessions with mother and infant at which mother is shown how to show love.

4   After ten sessions mother shows love towards the child.

5   Professional considers cause has been *cured*.

6   Infant still regularly soils and smears faeces over bedroom wall.

The behavioural view avoids the difficulties associated with searching for internal causes by taking a problem-centred approach: the problem—and not some imagined cause—is dealt with directly.

The general idea of the behavioural view

The behavioural view says we behave as we do (for example not stealing, not hitting others, not spitting in dining rooms, not going about naked and so on) because we have *learned* to behave this way.

From a very early age individuals begin to learn what behaviours society finds acceptable and unacceptable through rewards and punishments given when behaviour occurs. Different societies have different standards and rewards and punishments are applied accordingly.

The most important period of this kind of learning is childhood. Gradually society's standards become internalised and an individual becomes his or her own source of rewards and punishments; for example congratulating him or herself for being polite and feeling guilty for being rude. How this comes about is briefly described next.

The theoretical background

Learning theory says that people behave in the way they do because of their past learning experiences, and that learning can be organised and planned to produce and eliminate particular behaviours. It is the most unified, coherent and long-lived theory in psychology. Its present form dates from the 1920s and since then it has been tested and explored rigorously (though not without problems).

There are three major strands of learning theory. They take different routes but employ the same learning principles. Learning theory has grown out of these strands.

1 Classical conditioning

This is concerned with reflexes which are caused by particular events or things: for example, a loud noise elicits a jump. The noise is an unconditioned stimulus (UCS) and the start is an unconditioned response (UCR). They are called 'unconditioned' because they don't have to be learned. Classical conditioning shows how this natural connection can develop with learning. For example, if the loud noise is repeatedly paired with a neutral stimulus, such as a red light, after a while the red light flashed alone will elicit a jump. The red light is now a conditioned stimulus (CS) and the jump response to it is a conditioned response (CR). These are called 'conditioned' because they have been learned.

```
UCS————→UCR
(Noise)      (Jump)
 ↓ ↓ ↓ ↓
CS ———→CR
(Light)      (Jump)
```

This diagram shows what happens if a red light is flashed every time a person is exposed to a sudden loud noise. After a time the light flash alone will produce a jump: the person has *learned* the jump behaviour.

Usually the CR is a weaker response than the UCR and it will 'wear out' over time if not periodically reinforced by pairing the UCS with the CS.

A person who has learned to jump to a red light may generalise that learning and jump when any coloured light is flashed. (This is called 'stimulus generalisation'). However, his jump will be stronger when the light is red. Thus he will vary his response. (This is called 'response generalisation'.)

You can see this type of learning in yourself. The words 'steak pie' will probably cause you to salivate. Of course the words alone cannot produce the effect. It is the complex connections you have learned over the years. Young children who have a history of being hit sometimes flinch when adults come too close. Again, this is a learned reflex. No doubt you can think of reflex behaviours you have learned in this way.

2 Operant conditioning

Classical conditioning deals with reflex behaviour over which a person has little control. When food is placed in your mouth, you cannot choose not to salivate. In other words, you cannot choose not to produce the behaviour. Operant conditioning deals with behaviour you choose to produce. For example, if the telephone rings you will probably answer it—but you do not have to. You can *choose* not to.

The process by which children learn to behave is largely a matter of operant learning. Young children produce lots of behaviours, some acceptable and some unacceptable in the society we live in. The acceptable ones are rewarded (or reinforced) and the unacceptable ones are punished. The purpose of this is to increase through rewards and punishments the number of times the child chooses to perform acceptable behaviour and not to perform unacceptable behaviour.

Parents and adults deal with children in this way automatically. For example, in any supermarket you will be able to see a parent criticising (punishing) a child for lifting a tin off a shelf and then praising (rewarding) the child for putting it back when told. This process takes place in thousands of situations with different behaviours and over time the child learns the standards for our society.

In older children who are badly behaved, operant learning tells us they are choosing not to produce wanted behaviour. They must then be taught to choose to produce wanted behaviour more often through the use of rewards and punishments. For example, a 14-year-old who gets out of his seat in class must be taught, with rewards, that staying in his seat is worth choosing and, with punishments, that getting out of his seat is not worth choosing. If this is applied systematically, the frequency with which the 14-year-old chooses to stay in his seat will increase.

3 Social learning theory

Social learning says that unacceptable behaviour (such as tantrums) is a consequence of faulty learning (through operant processes), and that it should be tackled by the input of correct learning through operant processes. Faulty learning, however, need not be inefficient learning. For example: a child who regularly receives from his mother the privilege that his father has refused him learns very quickly to 'go behind his father's back'. Another child, whose bullying ways are thought of as 'manly' by his father will learn efficiently to hit others whenever he wants. As time goes by children will respond to the consistency of the lesson and come to believe that this is right for them; the lesson is internalised. The process has been efficient but the message has faulty content.

Now answer the following questions:

Question 1 List three rewards that operate in your life.

Question 2 List two behaviour problems that are the result of faulty learning.

Question 3 List three punishers (other than slaps, smacks and hitting the child) that children dislike.

INSTRUCTOR 7

The material covered in Handout 2 is best dealt with section by section. Trainees are often surprised to find the theory so straightforward. Some, however, will not like the simplicity. But this handout is not a basis for a philosophical argument: its purpose is to summarise the core concepts in the behavioural view.

Possible answers for the questions in Handout 2:

1   Three rewards that operate in most adults' lives include:

(a) The cheque at the end of the month.

(b) Praise from others.

(c) A cup of tea self-rewarded at the end of a tiresome task.

And there are lots of others, of course.

2   Any two behaviours that clearly have been acquired by faulty learning.

They may include destruction of parents' belongings, stealing money to buy friendship, truanting to avoid failure at school, 'heart-broken' sobbing to ward off punishment, snatching toys from other children, telling lies to avoid punishment.

3   Three punishers (other than physical punishers) may include:

(a) Not being able to watch a favourite TV programme.

(b) Not being given money for sweets.

(c) Having to tell a teacher you have been naughty at home.

And there are lots of others.

The nature of learned infant behaviour problems

Using the behavioural framework given in Handout 2, we can broadly differentiate three varieties of maladaptive behaviour from infants.

FAULTY NEW LEARNING   Many problem behaviours are learned in the same way that 'good' behaviours are. Faulty learning occurs because the first instances of it were inappropriately reinforced by the parents or other caretakers of the child. For instance one little boy started banging an oven door loudly, something he had not done before, and his grandmother looked at him delightedly saying 'Look, Ricky is playing the drums—give us a nice tune'. Subsequently she inappropriately rewarded this behaviour by saying 'Drums again!—I'll get some for Christmas'. She positively reinforced this new behaviour making it more likely to be repeated to the point where it became a problem.

PERPETUATED
EARLY
BEHAVIOUR

From the earliest point of development babies express the discomfort of hunger, wetness, boredom or whatever by crying and, if ignored, screaming with bodily gyrations. They are totally egocentric and their parents normally respond to this behaviour as quickly as they can. Gradually, however, parents become annoyed by these embryonic tantrums and require more mature forms of communication such as gestures and eventually speech.

This normal pattern of development, however, can be delayed by poor management or parents' inability to stop themselves responding to crying and screaming. Temper tantrums are the end result and represent the classic example of perpetuation of immaturity by a failure to stop the 'reward' of attention that maintains such behaviour.

BEHAVIOURS
AGGRAVATED BY
BIOLOGICAL
CONDITIONS

Examples of these include autistic behaviours, temporal lobe epileptic personalities, fragile X syndrome behaviours, and so on. These constitute less than 1% of disturbing infant behaviour problems.

Fortunately, the first two types of maladaptive behaviour respond to more or less heavy doses of re-learning on a consistent and well structured basis. The third type requires such intervention but over a period of years, usually nearly into adolescence, and often there is never complete resolution. Behavioural interventions for this group, although long term and exhausting, are still more effective than 'medical' style approaches such as drugs, surgery, psychotherapy counselling and the like.

INSTRUCTOR 8

At this point we suggest a 15–10 minute discussion of infant behaviour problems. Encourage each trainee to cite an instance of maladaptive behaviour they have met and ask the whole group to discuss the way in which the child acquired it. Keep them to objective statements and re-remind them not to speculate on subjective reasons like 'emotional rejection', 'lack of love', etc.

Objective 3

To teach the effective analysis of behaviour problems

We have already introduced the notion of antecedents and consequences. It is now necessary to examine these in greater detail.

HANDOUT 3

The Wood family

Read the following story and then answer the questions at the end of it.

1 Mrs Wood has two children, John (aged 4 years) and Veronica
2 (aged 1½ years). They live in a tiny two-bedroomed council house. Her
3 husband left her for a job in the Arabian Gulf one year ago, and apart
4 from regular maintenance, neither she nor the children have heard from
5 him since.
6   Mrs Wood seems not to be too concerned about her separation but
7 she and her own mother are very worried by John's behaviour. He is
8 said to be hyperactive by the nursery staff and seems to show some
9 bizarre behaviour. At home he shows consistent management problems.
10 For example, his mother finds it almost impossible to prepare
11 Veronica's tea, which she likes to feed to the child, because John
12 empties cupboards upstairs, turns on taps, climbs on top of the
13 wardrobe, hangs from the banisters and shouts at the top of his voice.
14 His mother generally runs after him and eventually gets him to sit in
15 front of the TV with a snack in his hand.
16   At night, when Veronica is being washed in the kitchen sink, John
17 repeats his performance but more half-heartedly because he really
18 prefers to watch the TV while playing with his toys.
19   Mrs Wood spends about an hour each night when the children are
20 asleep talking about all this to her own mother. They are concerned that
21 John takes after his father, whose restless and roaming ways caused
22 him to live an almost gipsy existence before marriage. Part of the
23 telephone conversation dwells on their prediction of John's behaviour
24 when he wakes in the morning.
25   Mrs Wood knows that he will wake up about 7am and then get up and
26 go downstairs where he will pull out drawers, knock over ornaments,
27 scatter the contents of her food cupboards and climb on the table. She
28 is grateful that he does not wake Veronica. Mrs Wood has found that
29 John can be distracted from this early morning behaviour by food, so
30 that when she wakes up at about 7.30am she can put on the TV for him
31 (he likes the advertisements for toys) and give him crisps, peanuts and a
32 tin of Coke. This keeps him happy until it is time to go to the nursery by
33 which time she has cleared up the mess.

Now answer the following questions:

Question 1   List subjective comments given about John and any other family member.

Question 2   Define what you consider to be the worst problems (no more than three).

Question 3   List antecedents and consequences for the problems you have defined in question 2 above. Remember that antecedents are events that usually precede the problems and consequences usually follow them.

INSTRUCTOR 9

Ask the trainees to write their answers on a sheet of paper and hand it to you. Collate in the way described in Instructor 2 the general pattern of the responses and use these for discussion purposes.

Emphasise answers which match the criteria shown on the following text pages.

QUESTION 1   List the subjective comments about John.

Usable answers

Subjective comments about John:
'He is said to be *hyperactive* and seems to show *bizarre* behaviour' (lines 8 and 9).
Subjective comments about John's father:
'restless and roaming ways' (line 21).
'gipsy existence' (line 22).

Criteria

This is a 'revision' question—you will recall from Objective 1 the need for objectivity in the use of ABA. Once again the word 'hyperactivity' is used without a description of the behaviour that gave rise to its application. Similarly, 'bizarre' is someone's opinion based on their own assessment of undescribed behaviour. In the same way comments have been made about John's father.

QUESTION 2   Define what you consider to be the worst problems (no more than three).

Usable answers

(a)   John empties cupboards upstairs (line 12).

(b)   John turns on the tap when he should not (line 12).

(c)   John puts himself at risk by climbing on wardrobes (line 13).

(d)   John puts himself at risk by hanging from the bannister (line 13).

(e)   John shouts at the top of his voice when he should not (lines 13 and 14).

(f)   John pulls out drawers at 7am (line 26).

Criteria

Notice how these are problem definitions straight from the text and given in terms of observable behaviour. There are others; perhaps you can locate them.

QUESTION 3   List antecedents and consequences of the defined problems.

Usable answers

Let us take the usable answers (a)–(f) for Question 2 and determine what antecedents and consequences are known to us from the text.

(a)–(e) John empties cupboards upstairs, etc (lines 12–14).

Antecedents: Mum is making Veronica's tea while John is upstairs. The text implies that Veronica has tea separately from John as she is still fed by her mother.

Consequences: Mum generally runs after him (line 14).
She puts him in front of the TV (line 15).
She gives him a snack (line 15).

(f) John pulls out drawers, and so on at 7am (lines 26 and 27).

Antecedents: These are harder to determine from the text than those given above. We infer that he wakes up before his mother (who wakes around 7.30am). If this is the case (as would be revealed by questioning Mrs Wood) than an important antecedent could be lack of supervision at the time he wakes up.

Consequences: Mother distracts him with food (line 31).
She puts on the TV (line 30).
She gives him a tin of Coke (line 32).

Criteria

You will note that the criteria for these usable answers describe antecedents and consequences that are very close in time to the problem behaviours and can possibly be changed.

Explanation

These criteria do not imply that other longer term influences are not at work and we would have to accept that some of these influences are historical, in that they are inherent to probable 'weak' parenting skills from John's earliest life.

You may feel that other antecedents are important. For example, these could be added:

(a)   They live in a tiny council house that may be overcrowded (line 2).

(b)   The father left the family (line 3).

(c)   John has been without a father for one year (line 3).

(d)   Mrs Wood is pleased to see the back of the children's father, and may denigrate him in conversation with or overheard by John (possible inference from lines 21 and 22).

(e)   John's father was a 'restless and roaming man who preferred a gipsy existence' (lines 21 and 22).

However, why should any of these give rise to such habitual *and specific* problem behaviours? It is generally not useful to speculate that such time-removed antecedents are associated with bad behaviour.

As we cannot prove what has caused these specific problem behaviours and we cannot alter the marriage (or, probably, arrange for the family to be re-housed) it is necessary to stop thinking about causes altogether. Antecedents need not be causes of the behaviour but they help to maintain its regularity. The danger with these time-removed antecedents is that they come to be regarded as irremediable causes (which they are).

For this reason we consider only those antecedents and consequences which:

(a)   Are regularly close in time to the problem behaviour.

(b)   Can be changed in some way to see if behaviour change results.

In this way we are able to specify those antecedent events which may be encouraging the problem behaviour and those consequences which may be reinforcing it. We can then predict changes in the behaviour as consequences of changes in either the antecedents or consequences according to the laws of operant learning.

This kind of analysis is often called ABC

A for Antecedents

B for Behaviour

C for Consequences

HANDOUT 4

Using ABC No behavioural intervention can be designed properly until ABC analysis has been carried out for the problem behaviours under scrutiny.

It should be possible to identify antecedents and consequences for all behaviour, good and bad.

Try this example.

Antecedents	Behaviour	Consequences
I have a wife, five children and a gerbil to maintain.	I go to work.	I get a salary cheque at the end of the month.

Question 1 Now write down, in brief, details about two problem behaviours that you have encountered under the following column headlines.

Antecedents	Behaviour	Consequences

Your answers should specify an observable behaviour, antecedents which regularly closely precede this behaviour and consequences which regularly and closely follow this behaviour. Both antecedents and consequences should be open to systematic change.

HANDOUT 5

PART 1 TEST

Multiple choice test on Part 1

On Objective 1

1 A goal is:
(a) A method of dealing with behavioural problems.
(b) The cause of the behaviour problem.
(c) A statement of the desired change in behaviour.
(d) Both (a) and (b).

2 Problem behaviour should be defined:
(a) Using one's own expertise and experience.
(b) Objectively, in terms of what can be seen and/or heard.
(c) With sensitivity and compassion.
(d) By using a label.

3 Problems should be measured at the start because:
(a) Measuring is a good idea.
(b) Measuring tells you what the problem is.
(c) It helps parents come to terms with their difficulties.
(d) You can measure them later to see if there has been a change.

4 Problems must be:
(a) Observable and recordable.
(b) Describable and remediable.
(c) Both (a) and (b).
(d) Easy to deal with.

5 ABA (applied behaviour analysis) is:
(a) A method of examining behaviour problems.
(b) The same as ABC.
(c) A way of eliminating bad behaviour.
(d) A common cause of behaviour problems.

6 In trying to stop behaviour problems it is vitally important to consider:
(a) Relationships and attitudes in the family.
(b) The family's income.
(c) Conditions such as hyperactivity, autism and fragile X syndrome.
(d) None of these.

On Objective 2

7 The behavioural view says that:
(a) Problem behaviour is learned.
(b) It is useful to think of problem behaviour as being caused by things like diet and hyperactivity.
(c) Children who behave badly are rejecting adult values.
(d) Kind adults cause behaviour problems.

8 Rewards are:
(a) Far too easy for children to get nowadays.
(b) Things that stop children behaving badly.
(c) Anything that makes it more likely that a child will behave in a particular way.
(d) Things that a child ought to like.

35

9 Faulty learning means:
   (a) Children being rewarded for unacceptable behaviour.
   (b) Children being punished for acceptable behaviour.
   (c) Learning behaviour which is not acceptable in our society.
   (d) All of these.

10 Faulty learning is best corrected by:
   (a) Counselling the child.
   (b) Counselling the parents.
   (c) Unlearning the bad behaviour and re-learning good behaviour.
   (d) Finding a cause for the bad behaviour.

11 'Perpetuated early behaviour' means:
   (a) Children have not grown out of behaviours which were acceptable when they were much younger.
   (b) Problem behaviour (like tantrums) that last for hours.
   (c) Waking early in the morning and coming into parents' bed.
   (d) None of these.

On Objective 3

12 The antecedents to problem behaviour are:
   (a) Historical events that happened a long time ago.
   (b) Caused by parents' low intelligence.
   (c) Obvious.
   (d) Observable events that occur immediately before the problem behaviour occurs.

13 The consequences of problem behaviour are:
   (a) The observable things that happen to the child immediately after the problem behaviour occurs.
   (b) The observable things that the child does when he or she is behaving badly.
   (c) Always unpleasant.
   (d) The anger that parents feel.

14 When using ABC the first thing to do is:
   (a) B: Define the behaviour.
   (b) C: Determine the consequences of the behaviour.
   (c) A: Determine the antecedents to the behaviour.
   (d) Interview the child to find out why he or she behaves badly.

15 Which of the following is not a subjective statement:
   (a) 'John is restless and uncouth'.
   (b) 'John is an unhappy little boy'.
   (c) 'John is 4 feet tall'.
   (d) 'John releases his pent-up aggression by hitting his mother.'

Summary of Part 1

This part has covered three main areas. First it introduced the need for the objective definition of problem behaviour—that is, the specification of observable and recordable behaviour independent of the subjective information that frequently accompanies it.

Second the behavioural view of such behaviour was introduced along with the concept that in the context of intervention it is profitable to consider that all behaviour is learned. The resolution of problem behaviour must lie in the successful unlearning of such behaviours.

Third, the ABC method of behaviour analysis was introduced. Problem behaviours (B) are examined for regularly occurring antecedents (A) and consequences (C). The antecedents may serve to initiate the behaviour which can then be reinforced by the consequences. Intervention along behavioural lines is the manipulation of either (or both) antecedents or consequences.

Part 2 goes on to consider how these ideas and tools can be used to construct ways of changing behaviour.

Answers to multiple choice test on Part 1

1 (c)	6 (d)	11 (a)
2 (b)	7 (a)	12 (d)
3 (d)	8 (c)	13 (a)
4 (c)	9 (d)	14 (a)
5 (a)	10 (c)	15 (c)

Each correct response scores one point and trainees should obtain 13 points or more. A score of ten or less suggests that a revision of all Goal 1 material is needed. A score of 11–12 suggests that the relevant parts only be revised.

Further reading on Part 1

A. Bandura, *Social Learning Theory* (Englewood Cliffs, New Jersey: Prentice-Hall, 1977).
S. N. Haynes, *Principles of Behavioural Assessment* (New York: Gardner Press, 1978).
B. L. Hudson and G. MacDonald, *An Introduction to Behavioural Social Work* (London: Academic Press, 1986).
B. Sheldon, *Behaviour Modification* (London: Tavistock, 1982).

PART 2

To teach suitable methods of intervention
with the problem behaviours of young
children

This goal is subserved by three objectives:

1 To teach the use of contingent reinforcers and punishers.

2 To teach a set of specific techniques.

3 To introduce some methods of recording behaviour.

These are followed by a multiple choice questionnaire on Part 2.

Objective 1

To teach the use of contingent reinforcers and punishers

The solution to most infant behaviour problems lies in the consistent management of reinforcers and punishers. Desirable behaviour is rewarded (reinforced) and undesirable behaviour is punished. This section is about defining and delivering these.

Questions and answers

What are reinforcers and punishers?

Reinforcers are rewards given to strengthen desirable behaviour. That is their sole purpose—to strengthen desirable behaviour. Rewards are not just something a child likes, they actually cause the child to change its behaviour in order to earn them. In other words, if the behaviour doesn't change the supposed reward is not a reward at all.

Punishers are always effective in weakening undesirable behaviour. If the supposed punisher does not weaken a specified undesirable behaviour then it is not a punisher at all and so should not be used.

Sometimes supposed rewards and punishers do exactly the opposite to that which is intended.

In one instance a nursery teacher felt that she should praise a little boy every time he spoke to her. Her reason for this was that he was a very quiet child and seldom communicated with her. Ostensibly her idea was a good one, but she found that praise was, for that child, not a reward at all; in fact it led to his communicating with her less often. In other words, her 'reward' was actually a 'punisher' of the behaviour she wished to increase.

Similarly another teacher felt that she should give firm scolding to an extremely active young boy who continually left his place during story time. Her gentle requests for him to sit down met with only short term success but when she used this scolding method his behaviour became far worse. Her supposed punisher turned out to be an effective reward.

These examples, and many others like them, make it necessary for us to ensure that whatever reward we are offering a child actually leads to an increase in his desirable behaviour and whatever punishers we are offering actually lead to weakening of an undesirable behaviour.

What does contingent mean?

It means that the giving of the reward or punisher is dependent (ie contingent) on a specific behaviour first occurring. The reward is given *only* if a desirable behaviour occurs and the punisher is given *only* if undesirable behaviour occurs.

Can contingent rewards and punishers be used within the same intervention?

Yes. The following example shows this working.

Joanne was 4 years old and attended a private nursery in a private housing estate within a large city.

At home she was very difficult to manage being given to severe tantrums involving screaming, followed by breath holding, throwing objects, overturning furniture, vomiting deliberately and lashing out at anyone within reach. These difficulties occurred only at home. The parents agreed that the priority problem was temper tantrums which always occurred after refusal of Joanne's demands. Parents gave in immediately and the child got exactly what she wanted! The parents were therefore giving a reward *contingent* upon Joanne's production of the undesirable behaviours. It was observed that Joanne's temper tantrums always began with shrill screaming, the other behaviours followed on as she got 'into the swing of it'. Applying ABC to this:

Antecedents, Joanne demands something; parents deny it.
Behaviour, Joanne starts screaming.
Consequences, Parents give her what she wants.

A simple scheme was devised to overcome these difficulties.

(a)   The parents would never give Joanne anything (from a list of non-essentials) that she asked for.

(b)   As soon as the screaming started she was taken to her room without comment, where she was left.

(c)   If she came out still screaming, she was returned, again without comment.

(d)   If, within 5 minutes of a want demand being refused, Joanne had not started screaming (or any other tantrum behaviour), she was rewarded with praise and either a toy or a sweet from a reward 'menu' kept for that purpose.

(e)   Whenever Joanne completed a task requested by one or other parent without complaint she was rewarded from the same reward 'menu'.

This procedure enabled rewards and punishers to be given contingently within the intervention and ensured that there was little risk of reinforcing unwanted behaviour.

Records kept of screaming frequency showed that there was an initial increase as Joanne 'worked harder' to re-establish her dominance. Within 7 weeks however, the problem was significantly reduced.

Do rewards always have to be given?

We should always try to fade out rewards. Praise, however, is not something that we need to phase out, it is relatively easy and 'cheap' to give and constantly reminds the child that his desirable behaviour leaves him in a state of grace.

What does praise entail?

The giving of praise should follow three rules.

(a)   Many people find it hard to praise children for behaviour they believe should be displayed anyway. Consequently they sound stilted and reluctant and rob what they say of much reward value. So the first rule is:

PRAISE MUST SOUND ENTHUSIASTIC

(b)   The second rule concerns immediacy. Where the child is being praised for new behaviour it should be rewarded immediately. If not, the child may start to do something else (scratch, look out of the window, fidget and so on). The praise reward, when it comes, reinforces this inserted, undesirable behaviour. The second rule is:

PRAISE SHOULD BE GIVEN AS SOON AS THE GOOD BEHAVIOUR IS OBSERVED

(c)   The praise reward should remind the child of the good behaviour. The adult should not say, for example, 'Good girl, aren't you lovely and clever!'. Instead the adult should specify what the child did that was good: 'Good girl for putting your toys away'. The third rule is:

ALWAYS SPECIFY THE BEHAVIOUR IN THE PRAISE STATEMENT

What if the child gets bored with the reward?

This happens in those circumstances where a reward 'menu' has not been planned.
   A reward 'menu' is simply a list of interchangeable rewards which can be used to provide a varied diet to maintain interest.

What sort of things go into a reward menu?

In order to construct a list it is a good idea to separate rewards under three headings: consumable, social and activity rewards. You can use these headings to generate ideas.

Consumable

Small sweeties
Crisps
Any food enjoyed by the child that can be given in small 'pieces' for example: yoghurt, cheese, biscuits.
Any drink that can be easily given in small quantities

Social

PRAISE
Pats, cuddles,
Tickles, bounces on knees

Star charts
Tokens
Pocket money
Smiling faces drawn on a card
Nice notes to/from nursery school
Special letters from grandma/father
Interaction over story book/bedtime

Activity

Play with a favourite toy
Special play in the bath
Model making
Cutting/colouring with parents
Dressing up special happy toys
Riding bike with Dad
Pouring water in and out of containers
Extended TV rights

What sort of punishers can be used?

Professional people should not advise parents to use physical punishments.
The types we can discuss generally involve the removal of rewarding
events or objects from the child or the removal of the child from them.

Examples
Response cost. This means that removal of the event or object prevents the
child from responding to it in a pleasant and rewarding way.
Time out is another example of punishment as removal of rewarding
events.

Antecedent 1	Antecedent 2	Behaviour	Consequence
The family is happily eating the evening meal	Mother says 'Stop playing with your fork, Joanne'	Joanne throws her plate on the floor	Joanne is immediately put outside the room and prevented from coming back in

In this example it is impossible to punish Joanne by removing a rewarding event or object—she has
already 'removed' her food and plate! Thus she has to be removed (time out) from the pleasant
situation of being with her family.

Antecedent	Behaviour	Consequences
Parents go to bed	Robert immediately leaves his bed and tries to get into theirs	Robert is instantly returned to his own bed

In this example Robert is being removed from a highly specific type of reward—the pleasure of being in bed with his mum and dad. The punisher used here is designed to *extinguish* the undesirable behaviour.

The most common example of time out has been used by generations of parents.

Antecedent 1	Antecedent 2	Behaviour	Consequence 1	Consequence 2
Mary wants X	Mother denies it	Mary whines and whimpers	Mother starts to talk her out of it (rewarding)	Mother gives her a cuddle (big reward)

The situation changed to the following during intervention:

Antecedent 1	Antecedent 2	Behaviour	Consequence
Mary wants X	Mother denies it	Mary whines and whimpers	Mother turns away and says nothing at all to Mary (extinction).

INSTRUCTOR 10

Handout 6 has three short case histories, each followed by one or more questions related to contingent reinforcers. The accompanying text pages explore these questions and give definite answers as a basis for discussion.

Instructors can choose either to discuss trainee's answers and the provided answers one story at a time or they can choose to ask the trainees to complete all three stories before discussion. Either way, the 'golden rules' illustrated must be stressed.

The same applies to Handout 7 which has two case histories with questions related to contingent punishers.

HANDOUT 6

'Golden rules' for rewards
Read these stories and try to answer the questions as briefly as possible.

Stefan
Stefan was nearly 4 years old when his desperate mother referred herself to the child guidance centre. He was very tiring for her and her priority behaviour problem was his wandering off when her back was turned during housework. It was noted that Stefan did not play with his toys for more than a few seconds before leaving them, so she was advised to reward him for playing longer (so that he would have less time for wandering out of the house). Accordingly his mother told him that he would get an extra sweet at lunchtime and another after tea for spending longer with his toys. Also, if, by the end of the day, he had not left the house without her permission, she would read an extra long story to him. The professional dealing with Stefan's case felt that his mother, who had generated these ideas herself, had really understood the technique very well.

Question 1 In your opinion, what is the main problem with the method described above?

Question 2 How would you improve it?

Gareth
Gareth was a 3-year-old boy with Down's syndrome. He was being trained by his mother to eat with a spoon. She intended to reward him with sips of his favourite 'pop' from a mug every time he managed to get the spoon to his mouth. Unfortunately, she quickly gave up this approach because Gareth kept tugging the mug handle after each drink, spilling lots of 'pop' over both of them and the floor.

Question 1 What has gone wrong here?

Darren
Darren, at age 4, had breath holding tantrums whenever he had to get dressed. His mother agreed that he could always play with a particular set of toys immediately after getting dressed, provided he threw no tantrums. She was supposed, therefore, to praise him and then follow this with the instruction 'You can play with your X now' (where X was the toy). On occasions, however, she was observed to say very quietly 'Good boy, off you go and play now'. At these times Darren looked puzzled, and began to look away from her obviously not attending to the situation at all.

Question 1 What is happening here?

'Golden rules' for rewards

STEFAN   *Question 1*

The major problem is the probable delay built into the giving of the reward.

Although adults can wait for an expected reward, for example until the end of the month for their salary, pre-school children cannot wait for even a few hours.

By the time Stefan gets his sweet all sorts of behaviour will have come and gone—some of it will almost certainly be undesirable. For example, if he had played nicely until 10.30am, wandered off at 10.35am, kicked the dog at 11.00am and fallen downstairs at 11.45am, would it really be sensible to give him his sweet at 12 noon for earlier playing?

REWARDS SHOULD BE GIVEN IMMEDIATELY

Question 2

One possibility would be to start his play behaviour just before lunchtime so that there is less time for undesirable behaviour to creep in. A more effective approach, however, would simply divide the morning up into small time zones with the reward for playing nicely available at the end of each.

GARETH   His mother should not have had a full (or even half-full) mug or one with a handle. A half-inch of pop in the bottom of a wide mouthed beaker would have been far better. Many a good behavioural approach sinks without trace because of such tiny details.

REWARDS SHOULD BE EASY

DARREN   The main problem here is that his mother has not managed to gain Darren's attention to her signal that the reward is available. If this situation persists there will be no reward value at all. His mother was advised to make her signal much more definite—'You *are* a good boy for getting dressed nicely—you have a *good* game with your X now'. In this way she would be following the rules about enthusiastic praise of the specified behaviour.

INTENDED REWARDS MUST GAIN THE CHILD'S ATTENTION

'Golden rules' for punishers Read these stories and try to answer the questions as briefly as possible.

James James at 3½ years was a 'handful' to his mother. He would not listen to her instructions and caused a lot of damage by climbing on furniture and shelves, banging things with his toys, knocking down displays in shops, and so on. His mother tried to scold him but he took no notice. Eventually she would say, 'You wait until your Dad gets in'. His father typically arrived home at 5pm when James was usually playing or watching TV quietly. Dad was told how naughty James had been and then shouted at him and sent him to the bedroom. This pattern persisted for nearly six months before both parents began to realise that James' behaviour during the day was not improving and that he stopped playing as soon as he saw his father.

Question 1 What is wrong here?

Katy Katy was a 3½ year old girl with petit mal epilepsy and suspected mild mental handicap. She annoyed her father intensely by regularly wetting herself when he did not immediately attend to her. Apparently she often approached him with a picture book or toy to engage him in play with her. At times this was inappropriate (for example, when he was on the telephone, mending something or talking to a visitor). He tried to ignore her and then told her to go away. Katy then used to squat and urinate. He decided to smack her for this. He was pleased to note that this had the desired effect—she no longer wet herself. However, his wife pointed out that Katy seemed no longer to approach him for attention—instead she had began to play by herself in very stereotyped and restricted ways.

Question 1 What behaviour has been suppressed by the punishment?

Question 2 What has Katy learned?

Question 3 Could we redesign her father's response?

'Golden rules' for punishers

JAMES James is actually punished by his father for sitting quietly watching television. What is wrong is that the punishment is far removed from the problem behaviour it is intended to curb.

PUNISHMENT SHOULD BE GIVEN IMMEDIATELY

KATY *Question 1*

The smack has suppressed the wetting behaviour but has done so by suppressing one of the antecedents that led up to it, namely, an approach by Katy to her father. She has demonstrated a wellknown fact about physical punishment—it can lead to avoidance.

DO NOT USE PUNISHMENT THAT COULD LEAD TO AVOIDANCE OF DESIRED BEHAVIOUR

Question 2

Katy has not only learned to stay away from her father but has also learned to play by herself. Her developmental difficulties made this particularly bad for her as she could not generate imaginative 'healthy' play.

ENSURE THAT THE CHILD'S RESPONSE TO PUNISHMENT IS NOT MORE FAULTY LEARNING

Question 3

As we have noted before, punishment does not teach better behaviour. Basically Katy needs to learn to wait. Thus a better strategy to employ is one that teaches her to wait and rewards her for doing so.

PUNISHMENT OF UNDESIRABLE BEHAVIOUR SHOULD BE COMPLEMENTED BY THE TEACHING AND REWARDING OF APPROPRIATE BEHAVIOUR

Given these rules for punishment and those stated previously for rewards, you should now be able to re-design her father's response to Katy's problem behaviour. Use the ABC model:

Before changing father's response:

Antecedents 1, 2, etc   *Behaviour*   *Consequences 1, 2, etc*

Proposed changes to father's response:

Antecedents 1, 2, etc   *Behaviour*   *Consequences 1, 2, etc*

INSTRUCTOR 11

The trainees should be able to lay out a sequence of responses to this simple situation of Katy's. It might look something like this.

Before changing father's response

Antecedent 1	*Behaviour*	*Consequence 1*
Katy approaches father who ignores her.	Katy wets herself.	Father smacks her.
		Consequence 2
		Katy avoids father.
Antecedent 2		
Katy continues to distract him.		
Antecedent 3		
Father shouts 'Go away, Katy'.		

Possible changes of father's behaviour

Antecedent 1	*Behaviour*	*Consequence 1*
Katy approaches her father who smiles and says 'Wait please, Katy'.	Katy wets herself.	Father, holding her hands, makes her change her pants, and put the wet ones in a bucket or basin. He does not talk to her, smile at her or in any way make this pleasant.
Antecedent 2		
Katy continues to distract him.		
Antecedent 3		
Father says 'Wait. Don't wet yourself' and completes his task.		

Variations on this theme may be acceptable provided that they do not unwittingly reward the child for not waiting or wetting.

These simple changes to her father's response enable this mildly handicapped child to acquire the socially necessary ability to wait in a definite and positive manner. If the trainees understand these points they have mastered this objective.

Objective 2

To teach a set of specific techniques

There are several accepted techniques that may be used successfully to help manage and develop infant behaviour. Some of these are presented here through case studies which provide thorough examples of their use.

INSTRUCTOR   12

Familiarise yourself with the next two sections so that you can discuss them with the trainees in a chalk and talk fashion. To do this you have to have a good understanding of the materials.

In order to help you structure this teaching session, which need not last more than 20 minutes, give each of the trainees a copy of the next two handouts as they appear. The handouts contain the main points you need to make.

At the end of the session spend some time in free discussion about the method. This will enable you to determine whether there are any significant weaknesses of understanding. If there are, go over the relevant material.

HANDOUT 8

Techniques for teaching desirable behaviour

1 *Contingent reinforcement*

This refers to a process whereby a child is rewarded every time it completes a desirable behaviour. These rewards are selected from a pre-arranged 'reward menu'.

2 *Token economy*

This is a process of praise reward supplemented by the addition of 'tokens'. The child understands that these may be exchanged later for a big reward. The tokens are given only on completion of a specified desirable behaviour.

3 *Response competition*

This aims at rewarding a specified desirable behaviour which competes with undesirable behaviour. For example; a child cannot be swinging from the bannisters at the same time as earning a reward for sitting down and painting.

4 *Modelling*

The desirable behaviour is modelled deliberately and emphatically by the parent. The child is rewarded as soon as he/she manages to imitate all or part of the model.

5 *Shaping*

The behaviour to be learned is split up into smaller chunks, each of which is modelled and reinforced. Gradually bits are assembled and child's behaviour is 'shaped up'.

Techniques for teaching desirable behaviour

1 Contingent reinforcement

Each time the desired behaviour occurs the child is given a praise reward: 'good boy/girl', 'that's lovely sitting down'. This praise may be immediately followed by the giving of some other reward from the menu. Always give the praise first. The reason for this lies in a theory called secondary reinforcement which says that the praise will become associated with the more powerful extra reward and take on some of the strong reinforcing properties of that reward.

2 Token economy

Children of 4 years and upwards may be developed sufficiently for this technique to be effective. Basically they need to be able to understand the idea that 'tokens' may add up to a big reward. The notion is analogous to our understanding that we need to save up money in order to exchange it for something we wish to buy. The child is told that every time it completes a specified desirable behaviour it will earn a 'token'. When the child has gained a number of these it can exchange them for a rewarding object or activity. These 'tokens' can take many forms. Often they are multi-coloured stars stuck on a wall chart. Sometimes the 'tokens' are simple ticks on a little notebook, but they can be milk bottle tops or counters or spent matches kept in a little bag.

3 Response competition

This is a commonsense idea. It says a child cannot be misbehaving at the same time that he is behaving well. Consider this example:

Ricky was a 4-year-old whose behaviour at nursery had been described as 'hyperactive'. Eventually his mother was asked to remove him because the staff never managed to bring his behaviour under control; they found that he produced just too much undesirable behaviour for them to get to grips with. After only a minute of play or painting or whatever he should have been doing, he would leave his place, then snatch toys, kick children, overturn furniture and try to run out of the nursery. Other parents complained that he hurt their children and these complaints made the staff feel challenged and uneasy. Their responses had short-lived effectiveness in that they grabbed hold of him and tugged him back to his 'work' while scolding him loudly. He remained there briefly before another outbreak of trouble.

In such a case, it is hard to prioritise the most worrying behaviour but the ABC analysis provides some ideas.

Antecedent 1	Antecedent 2	Behaviour	Consequences
Ricky is told to do X (painting, brick building, etc)	Ricky gets restless after a few minutes	Ricky leaves his work, etc	As described above.

55

Ricky cannot snatch toys, kick others, overturn furniture and run out of the nursery if he remains in his place 'working', so the behaviour we should prioritise as being most undesirable is that of leaving his place—it is the antecedent for all the others. We can call this the priority problem behaviour (PB). The alternative, according to response competition is: 'Ricky will remain for longer periods in his place doing what he is supposed to'. We refer to this as the competing behaviour (CB).

Thereafter the intervention proceeds to reward gradually increased time spent working.

4 Modelling

Any child who is capable of imitating the behaviour of adults, albeit crudely, can be reached by this simple but effective technique. The parent 'models' the desirable behaviour that they wish the child to learn. The child's initial attempts to imitate this model should be rewarded no matter how poor these attempts may be. Gradually more and more refinement of the behaviour is required until the child is able to complete it without the model.

5 Shaping

Sometimes the behaviours to be learned are too complicated for the child to attain at once. Behaviour has to be shaped up, bit by bit until the child is able to complete the whole of it as one process. Generally speaking it is best to avoid complex behaviours with small children and parents but if they are unavoidable ensure that the parents know to break them down into small bits.

HANDOUT 9

Weakening undesirable behaviour

1 *Time out*

This is a process by which the child ceases to have available any rewards during or just after the production of undesirable behaviour.

The time out lasts only until the child has stopped the undesirable behaviour and has been quiet for a short time.

2 *Response cost*

A favourite object or activity is removed or denied the child immediately after the production of an undesirable behaviour. The child knows that he may only win the object or activity back by compliance.

3 *Restraint and guidance*

Restraint is used, after a warning, to bring about the end of undesirable behaviour. It must be given firmly and consistently but only by parents who are known not to become excessively angry or physical toward the child.

Techniques for weakening undesirable behaviour

1 TIME OUT   Time out is the method by which all rewards for undesirable behaviour are removed from the child or the child from them.

What form should the time out take?

We have already said that it can range from complete removal of the child to another room to simply turning one's face away from the child while silently ignoring it. How do we decide what to do within this range? The answer is always to try the simplest thing first. If it is possible simply to turn away and ignore, then try it, but if other small children or family members persist in making comments, smiling, and so on, then complete removal is necessary. If removing all possible rewards means turning off the TV or record player so that other people's enjoyment is affected then, again, total removal is necessary.

   If removal is decided on, it is then necessary to ensure that the place the child is removed to is both safe and boring. There should be no stairs to fall down or toys to play with. Some thought has to be given to what is possible and it may be that time out cannot be used. It is better to take this decision at the outset rather than have a poorly planned attempt backfire on the parents.

How long should time out last?

It should not be a fixed length sentence. The child must know how to win back the favour of its parents. Often this is a matter of stopping the time out as soon as all the crying, whining, foot stamping has ceased and the child is quiet again: 'You can come back when you are quiet' is the rule of the day. On other occasions where the time out has resulted from the child's angry refusal to do something, he or she can volunteer to do it properly and thus end the punishment. In these circumstances the child would not be rewarded for completing the task.

How does the child learn to do without time out?

He or she learns because the parents always give one (and only one) brief, sharp warning before time out is given, for example:

Behaviour	Consequence	Behaviour	Consequence
Child starts whining	'No don't whine' (looking directly into the child's eyes)	1 Child persists in whining *or* 2 Child stops whining	1 Time out starts 2 No further action

Notice that the warning is short and behaviour directed. It is not the commonly occurring long drawn out explanatory warning ('If you don't stop whining I'll get cross with you and then put you in time out until you stop'). It is also emphatically given in a raised voice with direct eye-contact so that the child knows it has been warned.

Gradually the pairing of this warning to time out leads to the warning itself acquiring some punishing properties. Thus the child learns to heed the warning and so do without the time out.

2 RESPONSE COST

This is a kind of fine involving the child in the loss of a favourite object or activity. There are some common problems with it.

Should the child lose the reward it earns for a desirable behaviour?

No. It may happen that the child is so naughty that it ends up never being rewarded for the desirable behaviour. This is the sure way to make the reward lose its reinforcing properties. Sometimes parents rip off stars from charts so often that the child never has enough to exchange for the big reward.

Does the child ever get the lost object or activity back?

Yes. The child must know how to win it back. Generally this means explaining what must be done: 'You can have the video back on when you have picked up your toys'.

How does the child learn to do without response cost?

The answer to this is as for time out; the characteristics of the warning are identical.

3 RESTRAINT AND GUIDANCE

These techniques often have rather arcane titles but in their simple forms, they boil down to physical restraint. Advocate them only if you are sure that the parents can complete them without loss of temper and possible physical risk to the child.

The first is simple restraint and an example was given earlier of parents returning Robert to his bed when he climbed into theirs. He was *restrained* from completing the undesirable behaviour of getting into their bed. Other examples are restraining a child from throwing bricks in a nursery, restraining another from overturning furniture and others from biting their wrists, head banging and the like.

How forceful should restraint be?

The amount of force required is that which immobilises the child without causing pain or physical damage. More often that not it merely involves holding an arm still. Or the child who will not, for example, remain in bed may need to be held there.

How long should restraint last?

As long as it takes the child to cease movement. This can be a matter of seconds but some children have been known to squirm or resist for as long as 30 minutes. Under these circumstances the parents need to be able to take over from each other so that it is the child who tires and not the parents.

How does the child learn to do without this type of punisher?

Again the warning is vital as it was for the last two techniques. It is also vital that a targeted desirable behaviour is taught to the child to compete with the punished behaviour. This last statement should be true for most punishment situations but it is particularly necessary with the restraint method. Thus the parents can reward more often than punish which will offset any of the avoidance side-effects of punishment that the restraint method may create.

The technique of guidance is often used by parents when a child refuses to comply with a request or instruction. For example:

Antecedents	Behaviour	Consequences	Behaviour	Consequences
'Sally put your toys away'	'Shan't—want to watch TV'	'No put your toys away'	1 'Won't' *or* 2 'OK' and does it	1 Child's limbs are firmly guided in putting toys away 2 No further action

Sometimes, with older children, it is often advocated that all refused instructions are dealt with this way but this is not always a good idea. Just because it is a necessary last resort for one refused instruction does not mean that it is necessary for another.

This form of guidance may be used where any instruction involving movement is refused; not tidying up is an obvious one, and failing to put on clothes, replacing knocked over objects are all suitable for the guidance of a child's limb to complete the instructed task.

Why does guidance act as a punisher since a child may enjoy the contact it brings?

Most children hate it. While it is not physically painful it is certainly psychologically aversive. Their willpower and control over their own bodies are undermined. But some children do enjoy the process. Their smiles and chuckles should instantly alert the parents who must stop using this method immediately.

How does the child learn to heed the warning?

Again, the answer lies in the firm sharp warning *but* take notice of the difference in the warning given before guidance starts and those warnings given before the other methods are used. The example about Sally shows clearly that the warning takes the form of a repeated instruction, said firmly, using the same words as originally used. This is necessary in order that the child associates the guidance with the instruction. We do not want the child to rely on guidance for all instructions indiscriminately.

INSTRUCTOR 13

The next handout contains two short case histories. They should be dealt with one at a time using the subsequent text pages.

Story 1 Chris.

There are no questions to go with this story. In group (whole or part) discussion, trainees should be asked to provide an ABC analysis of the problem and then go on to explore the main points of a possible intervention and the notion of response competition, punishers and rewards to weaken and strengthen behaviours respectively. The accompanying text pages provide a framework of points within which this discussion can be directed. Use of an overhead projector is advised.

Story 2 Kim.

For the four questions that go with this, sample answers are provided on the accompanying text pages. Using an overhead projector, instructors may elicit a range of answers to each question and then compare these with the samples provided. To be 'right' the trainees' answers need not be the same as the samples, but they should follow the same criteria.

It may be the case that experienced instructors choose not to use the text pages. The trainees' responses, with guidance, may provide enough sound material for discussion as long as they cover the main points of the text.

HANDOUT 10

The techniques in practice

Chris   Chris was nearly 5 years old and had just entered his infant reception class. Despite being a loving child, fond of his parents' and teacher's attention, he had serious temper tantrums at both home and school. He would lie on the floor, shouting, screaming and banging his feet. Despite the fact that both mother and teacher said that he was always like this, it happened on average three times a day only after he was asked to do something other than play by himself. Somehow he had learned that tantrums enabled him to avoid work.

Kim   Kim was a 4½ year old tyrant queen! Since the birth of her baby brother she had turned really nasty. On one occasion she threw him on the floor and on another she had deliberately broken his toys. She never did what her mother asked of her although she was good for her father. Kim was also very destructive of any property not her own. In addition she was twice caught climbing out of windows and on one occasion got into her mother's car and slashed the roof with a knife taken from the kitchen. She wore her parents out by nightly refusing to go to bed until they did; whereupon she would sleep normally. Kim was eventually seen by a psychiatrist and the latter told the parents she was going through a phase of sibling rivalry which she would eventually grow out of. Unfortunately the nerves of her parents couldn't wait that long!

The most persistent difficulty occurred whenever her mother fed the baby. Then Kim strewed the contents of drawers, toy boxes, magazine racks and book shelves over the floor. Afterwards, as her mother got on hands and knees to pick the objects up, Kim repeatedly climbed on her back and insisted she played 'horsey'. Her mother gave in to this demand because otherwise Kim had bad tantrums during which she had once broken a glass dividing door and on another occasion a dining chair.

Question 1   Underline three subjective red-herrings.

Question 2   Write down one priority behaviour for intervention.

Question 3   Why have you selected this priority behaviour.

Question 4   Design the framework of an intervention that employs response competition.

The techniques in practice

CHRIS   *Response competition* can be used to define an alternative behaviour. In this instance the PB is the tantrum behaviour—this must be weakened or removed entirely. The CB must somehow involve obedience to instruction on the grounds that Chris cannot have a tantrum while doing as he is told.

We already know that the PB occurs on average three times a day, when a set task interferes with playing by himself. During the course of a school day there will be many more instructions than this; obviously, therefore, he obeys most of these (or at least does not have tantrums after hearing them). What is the difference between instructions which initiate tantrums and those which do not? Discussion with both parents and teacher using ABC should reveal the answer.

Antecedent 1	Antecedent 2	Behaviour	Consequence
Chris is playing by himself	'Chris, please do X' (where X is a task)	Chris has tantrums	After cooling down he is able to return to play by himself

This is a common situation. Many parents and teachers back down in the face of a massive tantrum. The child gets hot and blotchy, sweating and distressed, sometimes tearful. Even if the adults do not try to talk the child out of it, they may not persist with their request. In this instance Chris gets the reward of going back to playing by himself

The notion of response competition has been used here to provide a framework for an intervention. So we now have:

1   A behaviour, tantrums, to weaken by means of punishers (the PB).

2   A behaviour, doing as told, to strengthen by means of rewards (the CB).

1 Weakening the PB

Time out was used whenever Chris had a tantrum. At home this meant putting him out into the hall of the bungalow (where there were no stairs). At school it meant he was made to sit isolated in a 'naughty chair' at the front of the class facing the wall.

2 Strengthening the CB

Token economy was used whenever Chris obeyed an instruction given in a situation (such as playing by himself) where he was inclined to have a tantrum rather than comply. Ten tokens meant a bike ride round the park with one of his parents.

It is not, of course, possible to separate these intended rewards and punishers into discrete, self-contained, categories. The time out, once it has been experienced, can serve to strengthen the CB because its absence can be rewarding. Similarly, the absence of tokens for tantrums can serve to weaken the PB.

KIM *Question 1*

Subjective red-herrings include:

'she has turned really nasty'

'she never did what her mother asked of her' (most unlikely)

'a phase of sibling rivalry' (anybody could guess that, so what?)

Question 2

The priority selected was the daily strewing of articles which her mother had to pick up.

Question 3

This priority was selected because Kim's mother became totally subjugated by her daughter as a consequence of the game of 'horsey'. Not only had she lost control of her daughter's behaviour but Kim was rubbing salt into the wound by insisting on this game. Kim was demonstrating her ability to control her mother's behaviour.

Question 4

The intervention finally used employed the response competition methodology supported by contingent reinforcement as reward and guidance and time out as punishment.

Kim was told to do something while the baby was being fed. If she did so then she was immediately rewarded (praise and sweets or a game). If she started to strew the floor with objects she received a firm warning then, if she persisted, her mother took her wrists and made her pick up and replace each object. All attempted tantrum behaviour was ignored.

Progress was recorded by simply counting the number of times Kim did as she was told.

The activities Kim was told to engage in were pre-selected by her mother from a range of things that Kim could do over a period of 10 minutes or so. Furthermore it was suggested to her mother that Kim's activity and feeding the baby always took place in the same room so that her mother could provide verbal prompts and on-going comments. Kim's mother took this idea further by making some of the activities given to Kim those that would involve her helpfully with the baby.

For the first week Kim's behaviour was really difficult. The second and third weeks saw a steady improvement.

Objective 3

To teach the use of methods of recording

This is a brief section because, although there are many complicated methods of recording behaviour the simplest are generally quite sufficient. There is seldom any need for anything more complex than simple ticks on diary pages.

Three major types of behaviour records—frequency counts, duration and timing—are described. As in previous sections recording methods are illustrated through case work examples. Finally there is a section on the effects of some interventions on some behaviours as revealed by the parents' records.

INSTRUCTOR 14

Instructors may complete the following text pages in a chalk and talk way stressing the 'golden rules' for each broad category of measurement type. There are many possible permutations of these three categories and discussion on this should be encouraged. Moreover, there are a number of other types of measurement, such as time sampling, which because of their more specific nature are not included here. However, whether or not instructors choose to expand and include will depend on the needs of particular groups of trainees: generally, more experienced trainees are equipped for the more sophisticated recording devices. The handout which follows the text gives examples of the three categories of measurement in action. Use of these categories for these examples is not final and trainees should be encouraged to explore other possibilities provided they match the criteria for measurement.

The final text page is a warning about measurement and this should be discussed by the group.

Major criteria for record keeping

SIMPLICITY Whatever recording system is used it must be simple to operate and involve a minimum of effort. A system that is too complex and time consuming encourages errors, undermines enthusiasm and can wreck potentially effective intervention plans.

REPLICABILITY   Any recording system must be capable of being repeated in exactly the same form on future dates. Recording is an index of whether or not the method of intervention is effective over time and, in turn, of whether or not the child's behaviour is changing—be it for better or worse. If the recording system changes from time to time these questions cannot be answered because even slightly different recording systems can be measuring completely different behaviours.

OBJECTIVITY   Records must not be based on the measurement of subjective impressions such as the number of times parents felt depressed about their child's behaviour. If it is to have any practical value a recording system must be concerned with measuring observable behaviour.

Three main categories of measurement

FREQUENCY   These are the most frequently used records and involve making a mark
COUNTS   every time a specified behaviour is witnessed. Commonly they have to record two frequencies as most interventions employ response competition where it is desirable to record the frequency of both the undesirable prioritised behaviour and the competing behaviour.

   The types of behaviours that can be counted in this way are those that have an obvious beginning and end. This may seem like a fairly trivial point to make as all behaviours have a beginning and end—even sitting still doing nothing. However, some of these start and finish points are not obvious at all. For example, does watching the television start when we turn it on or when we sit down and face it? Does it end when we turn off the set or when we look away momentarily to accept a cup of tea being handed to us? This behaviour is really a continuous stream of behaviours. On the other hand making a cup of tea has an obvious start and finish. So does deliberately wetting the carpet or shouting angrily at mother, or refusing to go to bed. All these behaviours have clear beginnings and ends. These are discrete behaviours and all they require is a simple tick every time they are observed.

FREQUENCY COUNTS APPLY TO BEHAVIOURS THAT HAVE CLEAR START AND END POINTS.

DURATION   For behaviours which do not have obvious start and finish points,
RECORDS   watching television or paying attention to a lesson for example, it is more appropriate to measure the length of time they last. This involves noting when the specified behaviour starts, noting again when it ends and recording the time lapse.

   In these examples the measured behaviour is, most people would agree, desirable. (In other words, they are competing behaviours.) In such cases we expect the duration to *increase* if the intervention is being effective.

   Measurements of duration can also apply to behaviours for which a start and end can be easily identified. Application of duration measurements to discrete behaviours is most appropriate where the behaviour in question happens relatively rarely, but each time lasts for several hours.

Imagine, for example, a problem of tantrums where each one lasted several hours. A frequency measure of, say, four times a week gives a misleading impression of the severity of the problem if each tantrum lasts for four hours. Moreover, a reduction of frequency from four to three following an intervention is equally likely to give a misleading impression of the efficacy of the intervention. It would be more realistic to measure the duration of the tantrums. In the case of these problem behaviours, the duration measure should *decrease* over time if the intervention is working.

DURATION MEASUREMENT APPLIES TO BEHAVIOURS THAT ARE NOT DISCRETE AND TO BEHAVIOURS THAT PERSIST CONTINUOUSLY OVER TIME.

TIMING   Time is appropriate where the child is required to do something at or by a particular time. Bedtimes are the classic example.

If the PB is identified as being that the child does not go to bed until very late, the most suitable way of setting a baseline is to note over a week or two the actual time the child does go to bed. This yields an average of number of hours and minutes late (beyone an ideal bedtime). The aim of the intervention would then be to reduce this average 'time late'.

TIME MEASUREMENTS ARE BEST USED WHERE FAILURE TO MATCH A DEADLINE IS AT THE ROOT OF A PB.

HANDOUT 11

**Examples of
recorded
behaviour**

Frequency

1 Kevin had tantrums. His mother had a note book with its pages divided
up into 1 inch squares for each day of the week. Every time he had a
tantrum she put a tick in the appropriate square. At the end of one week
she worked out the average number of ticks per square to give the
average number of tantrums per day. We call this first period of
recording the baseline which tells us how bad the problem is before
intervention starts.

2 Sally often refused to get out of bed to get ready for nursery and her
mother had to carry her out and then dress her. This was recorded over
a two week period. This represented a baseline taken over 10 (school)
days.

Duration

1 John could not concentrate on anything for very long but we were
unsure just how long he typically managed. During the course of a
week, his nursery teacher gave him a simple task once a day and noted
the time he spent on this task. At the end of the week she discovered he
worked for an averge of 1 minute at a time. This was his baseline result.

2 Mike regularly rocked his body back and forth. No matter what else he
was doing, he was rocking. His mother noted the start and end times of
each rocking session for every morning for one week. At the end of one
week she discovered that he rocked, on average, for 45 minutes at a
time.

3 Two-and-a-half-year-old Lindsay had acquired the habit of picking her
nose. She did this with great vigour at, seemingly, every opportunity.
She withdrew her finger when told but put it back in as soon as
possible. In order to set a baseline her parents set aside an hour each
evening for one week during which they did not tell Lindsay to stop, but
recorded the duration of each nose picking session *and the frequency*.
This baseline showed that on average Lindsay picked her nose three
times per hour for 2½ minutes at a time. Their aim was then to reduce
both frequency and duration.

Timing

1 Rachael seldom went to bed before 11pm. For most of the evening she
was tired and irritable and her ensuing behaviour caused considerable
disruption to family life. Her parents thought 7pm would be a suitable
bedtime. Over a period of two weeks they noted the time she went to
bed each night and calculated an average 'time late'. This turned out to
be 3¼ hours. The aim of their intervention was then to reduce this
figure gradually.

Some apparently worrying effects measurement can have

Recording behaviours can help parents discover that things are not as bad as they think. Others find things are worse but this is relatively rare. It can happen, however, that records kept during some interventions show a worsening trend.

Obviously it is necessary to maintain the records during the period of intervention. We have to know if we are being successful or not. These records can frighten parents because some behaviours are seen to get worse for a short period.

Many of the examples that we have given throughout this material have shown such a trend for a short period. Katy the tyrant queen got worse initially. When she found her mother was no longer giving her the attention she craved she worked harder to obtain it so she strewed more objects on the floor. For the first week she became much more difficult. Fortunately her mother had been told to expect this and the reason for it was explained.

In general, where the reward for an undesirable behaviour is withdrawn (such as the loss of attention) the child will work harder to regain the lost reward.

Do not be alarmed by this trend but always warn the parents that it is a possibility. In fact it is encouraging because such a trend means that the intervention is having an effect on the child.

HANDOUT 12

Multiple choice test on Part 2

On Objective 1

1 A reinforcer is:
(a) Rewards given to weaken behaviour.
(b) A punisher designed to strengthen a behaviour.
(c) Something intended to strengthen a behaviour.
(d) A reward that stops bad behaviour.

2 When praise is given, it:
(a) Must aim at the child personally.
(b) Should be given in a modest, restrained, deadpan way.
(c) Is always embarrassing for the child.
(d) Is none of these.

3 Punishment need mean no more than:
(a) One sweet instead of two.
(b) A good thrashing.
(c) Not getting a reward.
(d) A half-hearted cuddle.

4 Rewards should be given:
(a) When the child asks.
(b) Immediately the bad behaviour stops.
(c) When it is bedtime.
(d) Contingent on the child producing a specified 'good' behaviour.

5 Contingent rewards and punishments:
(a) Can be used within the same intervention.
(b) Cannot be used within the same intervention.
(c) Have exactly the same effect on behaviour.
(d) Have no effect unless the child enjoys them.

On Objective 2

6 Response competition:
(a) Means performing one behaviour robs the child of the opportunity to perform another.
(b) Is what happens when a child is confused.
(c) Involves giving the child tokens for behaving properly.
(d) Is a complex idea which can only be explained to parents with great difficulty.

7 Modelling is possible only if:
(a) The child is old enough to be able to mould Plasticene.
(b) The child is of at least average intelligence.
(c) A token economy had been tried first.
(d) None of these.

8 A token economy:
   (a) Teaches children the value of money.
   (b) Always involves sweets and money.
   (c) Is usually only suitable for children 4 years and over.
   (d) Always works.

9 Removing a child from a potentially rewarding situation is called:
   (a) Response cost.
   (b) Token economy.
   (c) Sending it to bed.
   (d) Time out.

10 In order to weaken behaviour parents should:
   (a) Supply 'punishment' when it occurs.
   (b) Reward all instances of good behaviour.
   (c) Bore the child.
   (d) Always use time out.

On Objective 3

11 Record keeping should always be:
   (a) Simple, replicable and objective.
   (b) Thorough, well presented and colourful.
   (c) Flexible so that it can take account of changing family circumstances over time.
   (d) None of these.

12 Counting the frequency of behaviours:
   (a) Is usually best left to experts.
   (b) Means noting the numbers of times each behaviour is witnessed.
   (c) Involves calculating how long problem behaviour lasts.
   (d) Should be done by the children themselves.

13 Duration measures are best suited when:
   (a) The behaviours concerned are discrete.
   (b) No other method of measurement can be applied.
   (c) The behaviour persists continuously over a period of time.
   (d) The problems have reached crisis point.

14 Setting a baseline for late bedtimes is best done by:
   (a) Time out.
   (b) The Kellerman system of measurement.
   (c) Noting the time at which the child appears tired.
   (d) Keeping a note of the times the child goes to bed.

15 Sometimes recording behaviour shows an increase in the problem because:
   (a) Recording is not perfect.
   (b) Having a reward for bad behaviour withdrawn makes the child work harder to get the reward back.
   (c) Children do not like having their behaviour recorded.
   (d) Recording makes children worse.

Summary of Part 2

Part 2 covered three central aspects of behavioural intervention. First, a number of rules were specified about the use of rewards and punishers and it was suggested that a reward 'menu' be drawn up for each intervention in order that the child does not become satiated by a single type of reward which could then lose its reinforcing properties.

Second a number of different methods for using rewards and punishers were described, stressing that it is rare to find interventions using only one or the other. Commonly, both are used consistently to help replace an undesirable behaviour with acceptable behaviour. The key concept here was response competition.

The third part dealt with the use of recording systems by parents and stress was laid on the need to keep things simple and objective. The key issue here is to establish the need for recording as the only accurate method of detecting change (good or bad) in a child's behaviour.

The next part aims to place this within an organised framework that can be delivered to families.

Answers to multiple choice test on Part 2

1 (c)	6 (a)	11 (a)
2 (d)	7 (d)	12 (b)
3 (c)	8 (c)	13 (c)
4 (d)	9 (d)	14 (d)
5 (a)	10 (a)	15 (b)

Trainees should obtain 13 points or more. Ten or less suggests revision is necessary. A score of 11–12 suggests the relevant parts only need be revised.

Further reading on Part 2

A. S. Bellack and M. Hersen, *Behaviour Modification: An Introductory Textbook* (Baltimore: Wilkins & Williams Co, 1977).
R. T. Butcher and K. E. Hewitt, *'If you don't believe'* ... *Practical Approaches for Parents and Professionals to the Behaviour of Young Children* (High Wycombe: Test Agency, 1986).
M. Herbert, *Behavioural Treatment of Children with Problems: A Practice Manual* (London: Academic Press, 1987).
E. C. S. Westmacott and R. S. Cameron, *Behaviour Can Change*.
(London: Macmillan Education, 1981).

PART 3

This goal is subserved by two objectives:

1 To teach ten steps to setting up a programme of intervention.

2 To provide an example of the ten steps in a real life situation.

It is important that you work through these in the order given before attempting the multiple choice questionnaire on Part 3.

Objective 1

To teach ten steps to setting up a programme of intervention

The objectives in Parts 1 and 2 provided a way of thinking about behavioural problems and a set of general methods for dealing with these problems.

Objective 1 here is more specific in that it concerns the way in which a programme for intervention, designed to correct a problem, can be derived and constructed. This is presented as a series of ten steps.

HANDOUT 13

Ten steps for constructing a programme of intervention

1 *Define the problem behaviours*

The details of this were given in Part 1.

2 *Choose a priority*

Children who present problems seldom, if ever, present only one problem. Attempts to correct problems often fail because adults try to solve all problems at once. The trap is easily avoided by selecting the problem the parents would most like to be rid of. Look for possible antecedents and consequences at this stage.

3 *Find a competing behaviour*

Nobody can be in two places at the same time. A child cannot be behaving badly if he or she is doing something else, hence 'a competing behaviour'. Finding a competing behaviour means finding an acceptable activity for the child to engage in which robs him or her of the opportunity to perform the defined problem behaviour. For example, the child who has been taught and has learned to make his babysitter laugh whenever he plays with her cannot also hit her over the head with a toy when he is playing with her. Similarly, a child who creates dangerous mayhem in the kitchen cannot do so if he or she is taught and learns never to enter the kitchen. These examples may be somewhat extreme: their purpose is to illustrate the point.

The exact nature of the competing behaviour will depend on what the priority problem is. However, it is vital that the competing behaviour be specified with the same objectivity as the problem behaviour.

4 *Set baselines*

This means measuring, over a period of at least one week, the defined problem behaviour (PB) and the competing behaviour (CB). Some types of recording were discussed in Part 2. Two baselines are required: one for the PB and one for the CB. The baselines may amount to no more than the total number of times each behaviour is noticed in a one hour session every day for a week. Thus the baselines might be: PB = 36 times per week, CB = twice per week.

5 *Determine rewards* (and punishers, where appropriate)

In Part 2 a reward was defined as anything that a child will change behaviour to have. Different children respond to different rewards. So for any child, a unique list—or menu—must be set up. This can only be done with the parents' help. Actions to be taken when the unwanted behaviour occurs must also be determined (punishers). This may be no more than not getting a reward.

6   *Design a method of intervention*

Based on what the PB is and what is known about its antecedents and consequences, design a method of delivering these rewards (and of withholding them) on a contingent and consistent basis: that is whenever CB and PB appear. The programme should be guided by the general principles given in Part 2 but these are flexible enough to allow modification to suit different families' individual needs.

7   *Maintain the recording system*

Whatever recording system was used by the parents to set the baseline should be maintained during the period of intervention. This period of initial intervention should not be less than 3 weeks.

8   *Go back to baselines*

After at least 3 weeks the intervention programme should stop and the baselines be measured again for a period of one week. This is for comparison with the first baseline set.

9   *Modify or maintain*

If there is no significant difference between the two baselines (ie if the CB has not increased and the PB has not decreased) then the method of intervention is not working. If this happens, the method needs to be closely examined and modified as necessary.

But if there is a significant improvement then the programme can be continued until the problem reaches an acceptable level.

10 *Discuss*

It is all too easy to carry out this procedure in a vacuum and to forget that this is part of a parent training process which, we hope, will equip them with skills they can use with other problems. Consequently the professional should discuss what has happened with the parents and make quite certain they know exactly why they have been advised to adopt certain practices.

INSTRUCTOR 15

The last handout summarises for the trainees the ten steps for intervention. These steps invariably raise questions, the most common of which is: 'This looks very time-consuming. I just don't have that much time.'

It is important to stress that the steps outline what is happening but not who is doing what. The professional's role is necessarily at the supervisory and organisational level, guiding the parents by offering them techniques and skills to use themselves. For example, while it is the professional who advises on methods of setting a baseline, it is the parents who actually observe, count and note the occurrence of the defined problem.

The text that follows expands on the details of each of the ten steps. The instructor should distribute Handout 13, then go through the steps one at a time using the details in the text and asking the trainees to complete exercises where necessary. The details in the text also specify who (parents or professional) does what and about how long each step should take to complete with parents. The instructor should take every opportunity to stress the professional's advisory role.

Completing the steps

1   Define the problem behaviours (20 minutes)

This is a matter of talking with parents or other managing adults. The process will, initially at least, produce a list of vague concerns such as, 'There is something wrong with her', or 'He doesn't have much concentration', or 'She can be a right little so-and-so'.

In order for parents to express these worries, however, the child must at some time have produced actual behaviour. The task of the professional at this stage is to elucidate these behaviours.

Professional: 'What problems do you have?'
Parent: 'Well, he doesn't seem to know how to behave properly.'
Professional: 'What sort of things does he do?'
Parent: 'For one thing, he is violent with his toys.'
Professional: 'In what way?'
Parent: 'He doesn't play with them for more than 5 minutes before wanting to throw them at the wall.'
Professional: 'So one of your problems is that he throws toys?'

In this simplified example the process is gradually being refined until an agreed problem is reached. To agree other problems, the professional can ask, 'What other things does your child do?'

Mutual agreement on the defined problems is essential. There is nothing to be gained by attempting to force parents into accepting definitions of problems which they do not recognise as important or relevant, despite what you as a professional may think.

Inevitably, an occasion will come when parents do not accept a professional's view, even after considerable exploration and discussion, and when the professional feels he or she cannot compromise without undermining good practice.

If this happens then the parents have the right of way, so to speak. The family under discussion is theirs. They have asked for advice and exercised their right to reject it. At this point the contact should end. If they wish, the parents can ask advice from someone else.

Remember, too, that nothing is secret in this process. Everyone concerned should know exactly what they are there for—at this stage it is to define the problems.

INSTRUCTOR 16

There are a number of ways of using the dialogue between parent and professional.

1 Role play by instructors. The dialogue is a skeleton to be fleshed out. For example, it is a good idea for instructors to insert rambling unsolicited detail from the parent about what the child did yesterday at teatime. The instructor taking the part of the professional can then demonstrate how to keep bringing the discussion back to the point, the problems. If the dialogue is used in this way, then instructors playing parent roles are advised to throw in as many red herrings as they can.

2 Ask a trainee to take the role of the professional with the intention of trying to keep to the point.

3 Ask trainees to take both roles.

4 Alter the dialogue to demonstrate failure of parent and professional to agree on the problem behaviour. Then the role play can be pursued as in any of 1 to 3 above. Three things can be demonstrated to trainees here:

How to break contact gracefully.

How to break contact rudely.

How to use negotiating skills to avoid the need to break contact.

Whichever option is chosen, the trainees watching should be encouraged in a critical discussion.

---

2 *Choose a priority* (5 minutes)

Now you have a list of four or five objectively expressed problems. It is time to select one of them as a priority. Normally this is not a matter for negotiation: whichever one the parent picks is the priority.

However, you should point out to the parents any overlap between problems. Consider this list of problems.

(a) Child throws toys.

(b) Child has a tantrum whenever she does not get her own way.

(c) Child head-bangs.

(d) Child kicks her baby brother.

(e) Child screams when forced to do as told.

If parents were faced with this list which one would you advise them to choose as a priority? In most cases it would be (b). Why?

The answer is that it is likely that the other behaviours are part of the tantrum. If this is so, stopping (e) for example, will only cut one behaviour out of the tantrum. Stopping (b) by teaching the child to defer demands for immediate gratification, will, however, also stop all the other problems.

Whatever happens, only one priority should be selected. Remember, this is a training exercise for parents and it will fail if the task becomes too large to be manageable.

Now is the time to determine antecedents and consequences. Getting at these was dealt with in Part 2. Here it is only necessary to establish what they are and make a note of them.

3 *Find a competing behaviour* (10 minutes)

Behavioural approaches are very good at stopping problem behaviour. If all you aim to do is stop a problem behaviour then there is a strong chance you will be successful with that behaviour. However, there is an equally strong chance that the gap left will be filled with an entirely new—but just as unwanted—behaviour problem. (This is not to be confused with the notion of symptom substitution which is an entirely different concept and not in any way relevant to this material.)

The problem occurs because the child has not been taught and learned an alternative, desirable, behaviour to the PB. It is this alternative that is called the competing behaviour (CB). A CB is any behaviour which, if performed, robs a child of the opportunity to perform the PB.

Consider this example:

PB = Child has tantrum whenever he asks for a sweet (or something else) and does not get it.

CB = Child goes away quietly and plays with his toys when he is refused a sweet.

Clearly, the child cannot perform the PB and the CB at the same time. There are three main points to be noted about the CB.

1   It provides an opportunity for the child to get plenty of attention for being good. Previously, the surest way of getting plenty of attention was to be naughty.

2   It specifies for the managing adults when to give a lot of positive attention, and precisely the behaviour they are aiming to reinforce.

3   This process teaches the child what to do instead of the tantrum—that is, it teaches him or her a socially acceptable behaviour.

Notice that the CB has to be specified in the same objective term as the PB.

Now try the exercise in Handout 14.

HANDOUT 14

Competing behaviour

Here is a list of ten PBs. Try to generate a CB for each.

1 Child picks and peels wallpaper off the living room walls.

2 Child draws on walls with crayons.

3 Child removes all her clothes if left alone.

4 Child hits and kicks the cat whenever it is within reach.

5 Child bangs all toys repeatedly on the floor.

6 Child runs away and hides when she is called.

7 Child urinates on living room floor when he is left alone.

8 Child gets up at 5.30am every morning and switches on the electric fire and all the cooker rings.

9 Child screams, head bangs, hand bites and hits out when compelled to do something he does not want to do.

10 Child hits out at all visitors who come to the house.

INSTRUCTOR 17

Trainees will probably need a lot of guidance in completing the exercise in Handout 14 both because they are doing it without the benefit of parents and in order to keep their CBs both objective and closely related to the PBs.

There are a number of ways in which trainees can complete the exercise:

1 By individually supplying possible CBs to the instructor for discussion.

2 By arriving collectively at CBs through open discussion.

3 By an instructor taking the role of parent so that trainees can experience some problems of establishing practical and realistic CBs. This can be done with one trainee/one instructor or with one instructor in the role of parent and all trainees acting in consort.

No sample answers are provided for the exercise. This is because for each PB there is a very wide range of possible CBs. The main criteria are that CBs be:

1 Objective.

2 Practical.

3 In direct competition with the PBs.

4 Expressions of wanted, good behaviour.

4 Setting baselines (10 minutes to establish what the parents are to do)

The next task is to establish a means of setting baselines for both PB and CB. Some ways of setting baselines and measuring behaviour were discussed in Part 2.

Different types of behaviour are suited to different types of measurement. Tantrums may be best suited to a 'duration' type measurement (how long each one lasts) while swearing might be best suited to 'frequency' type measurement (how often it occurs). Problems of late bedtimes are best measured by recording the time the child goes to bed and soiling is best measured by frequency.

There are no hard and fast rules however. Any kind of measurement which gives some idea of the size of the problem is suitable. For example although duration is commonly measured for tantrums, this does not exclude the possibility of measures of frequency.

The three main things which a measurement device must have are:

1 Simplicity. It must involve the minimum of effort.

2 Replicability. It must be capable of being repeated at some later date.

3   Objectivity. It must not rely on the measurement of subjective impressions such as the number of times a child annoyed a parent; it must be concerned with observable behaviour.

You will gather from this that there is no list of measurement techniques. Measurement and baselining methods are best chosen to suit the individual situation, following the principles given in Part 2 and summarised in the three criteria above.

This section is concerned with the method of establishing baselines rather than with the details of measurement. Measurements of PB and CB should take place over at least one week (7 days). Thus the basic recording chart may look something like this:

Week beginning							
Days	1	2	3	4	5	6	7
PB							
CB							

The key features are:

(a)   Dating.

(b)   Spaces in which to record the PB and CB each day.

This simple chart should be seen as a skeleton from which more specific and detailed charts can be generated. How it might be developed to record different types of behaviour and different types of measurement is shown in Handout 15.

HANDOUT 15

Sample recording charts for different types of behaviour and measurement

1 *Hitting*

Week beginning							
Days	1	2	3	4	5	6	7
PB: Hits baby sister	⑭ /	///	////		//	⑭ //	////
CB: Makes baby sister smile	/					//	

This is a frequency count. Every time the parent has witnessed the PB or CB, he or she has entered a tally mark in the appropriate space.

2 *Tantrums*

The frequency count can also be used for tantrums (for example), in which case:

PB: Has tantrum when does not get own way.

CB: Accepts refusal and carries on as before.

Some people prefer to measure the duration of tantrums. In this case, reducing the length of the tantrums is the initial aim rather than stopping them. This is used mainly where tantrums are severe and where it is felt that stopping them altogether is too big a first step. For example:

Week beginning							
Days	1	2	3	4	5	6	7
PB: Duration of tantrums	30m	95m	10m	55m	12m		5m
CB: Plays quietly after tantrum	/	///					

3 *Running away*

Week beginning							
Days	1	2	3	4	5	6	7
PB: Runs away when called	///	⑭	//	/	////	//	///
CB: Comes after first call	/		///	/			//

85

4 *Bedtime*

Week beginning							
Days	1	2	3	4	5	6	7
PB: Time in bed	11.00	11.30	12.00	7.30	12.30	9.40	8.50
CB: In bed by 7.30pm				✓			

In this baseline you have a measure of the PB in terms of what time the child actually goes to bed. This allows the setting of realistic and gradual steps towards getting the child to bed at 7.30. If this baseline showed that on average the child was 4 hours later in going to bed, you know it would be unrealistic to start the intervention programme which *suddenly* requires him or her to go to bed at 7.30. This should be accomplished through a series of steps.

5 *Bedwetting*

Bedwetting baselines are best set over a period of at least 2 weeks because of the often intermittent nature of the problem. The record here is very simple.

Week beginning							
Days	1	2	3	4	5	6	7
Wet bed		✓		✓	✓	✓	✓	✓

The CB here would be 'dry bed', but it is not necessary—as is often the case—to record this separately since all the necessary information is obtained by recording wet days.

Once a method of measurement and recording is devised the chart should be drawn up at once. Doing it immediately has a number of advantages:

1   It allows the process of recording to start immediately.

2   It compels simplicity.

3   It allows parents to see that the process is not at all mysterious and that it is a device they can use themselves in future for other problems.

Since the records are to be completed by parents, you must be certain they know exactly what to do.

One of the main problems is that professionals often ask parents to keep the child under observation all day. This is usually impossible and it is likely to discourage parents. What we are seeking is a snapshot of the behaviour not an exhaustive record, although, since the method needs to be replicable some standards for recording must be set. This is best done by setting aside a period each day when observation and recording are carried out—perhaps a different hour each day. For example:

Week beginning							
Days	1	2	3	4	5	6	7
	9–10am	10–11am	11–12am	12–1pm	1–2pm	2–3pm	3–4pm
PB	///	### //	//	### ###	/	///	//
CB				/		//	

Obviously the times should be chosen to suit the circumstances. When the baseline is repeated at some later date, after the intervention programme, the same times must be used.

Observation does not mean that the parent has to drop everything and 'observe' the child. It should be stressed that they should carry on normally during the observation period; it is simply the time when the specified behaviours are recorded.

They should not look actively for these behaviours: rather they should wait till they come to their attention before recording them.

The final thing to do is to put the chart in the right place in the house. If the problem is one of bedwetting then the chart should go in the child's bedroom. If it is one of tantrums then the chart should go where the action usually happens—in living room or kitchen, for example.

THIS IS THE END OF THE FIRST STAGE AND THE FIRST VISIT. IT HAS TAKEN A TOTAL OF 45 MINUTES TO COMPLETE.

5 *Determining rewards*—and punishers where applicable (10 minutes).

It is surprising when parents are asked what their child likes how often they say 'Nothing at all!'. Since no child has no things they do not especially like, what parents really mean is that they (the parents) cannot think of anything.

The task of the professional is to help them to produce a list or menu of rewards. This might look something like this:

1 A Smartie.

2 Playing with Tonka truck.

3 Watching the Flintstones on TV.

4 Completing a jigsaw with Daddy.

5 Being cuddled and praised (positive attention).

There are several important points to bear in mind when setting up a reward menu:

1 The parents must specify these rewards.

2 Food rewards, if used at all, must be kept to an absolute minimum (half a Smartie is better than a whole one).

3 Things on the menu must not be available to the child at times other than when he or she is being rewarded. For example, if playing with the Tonka truck is a reward it must be kept out of reach at all other times.

4 Rewards chosen must be capable of being delivered immediately the CB is produced. It is pointless telling a toddler that if he does not hit his sister Mummy will play with him tomorrow.

5 'Punishment' may be no more than withdrawal of rewards. This is why it is important to accustom the child to being rewarded for good behaviour—punishment is knowing what he or she is missing. More active punishment, detailed in Part 2, should only be used with PB if a reward system is being used with the CB.

6 Whatever reward is delivered it must be accompanied by lavish amounts of praise and attention. Can you think of a reason why this is a good idea?

88

6 *Setting up a method of intervention* (30 minutes)

Essentially, this is a matter of determining the means of delivering rewards and punishers. Put another way, it is managing antecedents and consequences so as to effect change in behaviour.

The first thing to do is to consider the antecedents and consequences of the PB. If these are likely to be exacerbating the problem they must be removed, and the parents must be clear as to why.

In setting up a method of intervention the main problems you will face will be to do with consequences; rewarding, withholding rewards, and punishing.

1 It is likely that the child will be unaccustomed to being rewarded consistently for good behaviour (the CB in this case). Initially, then, the child might not be too bothered at having rewards withheld. To ensure that he or she does know what is being missed, it is important to provide as much consistent rewarding as possible for the CB.

2 Rewards are not to be confused with bribes. A reward becomes a bribe if when the child behaves badly (the PB), an adult tells him he can get a reward if he stops. This is teaching the child to behave badly. Rewards are for the CB, not for stopping behaving badly when asked.

3 Care should be taken with punishers to ensure that they do not become rewarding. To give any form of punishment to a child inevitably involves giving attention, which, for the children who get precious little attention, can be rewarding.

Parents should be absolutely clear on these three main points.

Other points that the intervention must stress are consistency and determination.

4 The CB must always be rewarded and rewards must always be withheld from the PB.

5 It is often very difficult to withhold any attention from a problem behaviour. The temptation to give a lot of negative attention over and above the agreed punisher can be overwhelming. This must be resisted. In the long run it does not work; if it did, the parents would not be asking for advice. Children who behave badly have had years to learn it. The problem is not going to be corrected overnight. Relearning is a longer, gradual process with ups and downs and it is all too easy just to give up.

At the end of this stage the parents should be clear on exactly what it is they are being advised to do. Inevitably there will be logistical problems: 'I can't do this part because ...'. It is because of things like this that delivering the intervention (and anything else) to parents is a matter of problem-solving negotiation. Only the parents can specify what they can and cannot do.

Whatever intervention you design, it must last for at least 3 weeks (preferably for 6 weeks).

7 Maintaining the recording system (5 minutes)

The recording system that was used for the baseline should be continued in exactly the same form. The only difference between this recording and the baseline is that there was no intervention taking place during the baseline.

If all goes well, the PB should diminish and the CB increase.

8 Going back to baselines (5 minutes)

Having decided how long the intervention is to last, ask the parents to run it for that time and then immediately return to the baseline condition. If, for example, the intervention is to run for six weeks, the parents should stop after that time and then repeat the baseline measurements in the same conditions as before. The results will indicate if the child is learning from the intervention. Suppose that the recording system maintained during the intervention shows a PB decrease and a CB increase. This looks as if the intervention is effective but it may be that the child is just responding to rewards rather than learning new behaviour. The second baseline will clarify this.

The second baseline may show no difference from the first in which case the child is not learning. It may show a significant improvement in which case you can conclude the child is learning.

Can you say why the intervention must be stopped for the second baseline?

It should take only 5 minutes to tell parents how to run the intervention for so many weeks and then return to the baseline. You should arrange a third visit for the time when the agreed schedule has been completed.

THIS IS THE END OF THE SECOND STAGE AND THE SECOND VISIT. IT HAS TAKEN A TOTAL OF 50 MINUTES TO COMPLETE.

9 Modifying or maintaining the intervention (40 minutes)

Where the two baselines show no significant difference it means one or more of the following have happened:

1 The intervention has been carried out improperly
Perhaps rewards have not been delivered and withheld consistently, or different behaviour has been rewarded. There are any number of things that could go wrong and the only way to discover them is to discuss with the parents exactly what they did.

2 There was a flaw in the intervention
For example, the rewards chosen were unsuitable in that the child did not value them enough or there was inconsistency because the PB was defined ambiguously. The whole process has to be reconsidered to identify possible errors.

3   The two baselines are not measuring the same behaviours
    This happens if the PB and CB definitions are ambiguous. For
    example, suppose the PB was 'Is violent towards baby sister' and on
    the first baseline this was measured as number of 'hitting' incidents.
    On the second baseline there is no reason in the definition why it
    should not be measured as the number of violent outbursts including
    shouting at baby sister to make her cry. These two baselines are not
    measuring the same behaviour and are next to useless as a comparison.

4   The intervention period has been too short
    All children learn at different rates. Some learn after one telling and
    others take a hundred tellings. If there is no problem with 1 to 3 above
    then run the intervention again and repeat the process.

Whatever fault or faults you discover, they must be corrected and the
process repeated.

Where the second baseline shows a significant improvement over the
first it is safe to assume that all is well. If this is the case go on to the next
step.

10   Discussing progress with parents (30 minutes)

If all has gone well, exactly what has happened should be discussed fully
with parents. The purpose of the intervention is not just to help parents
sort out a specific behaviour problem. You will have achieved very little if
parents sort problems one at a time and keep coming back to you for the
same advice for each one.

   The main purpose of the discussion is to establish that parents
understand behaviour good and bad is learned, that children can be
'untaught' the bad and taught the good, and that it is the parents who do
the teaching using the simple methods and techniques you have
demonstrated.

   They should now have learned:

1   Behaviour is learned.

2   How to define problem behaviour and competing behaviour.

3   Measurement of behaviour.

4   Intervention techniques and methods.

It is at this point you should decide on your future involvement. You
should keep uppermost in your mind the idea of minimum involvement so
as to avoid the problems of parents becoming too dependent on
professionals.

   It is preferable to arrange to visit in about 6 months' time for a general
discussion on how they are getting on.

THIS IS THE END OF THE THIRD STAGE AND THE THIRD
(POSSIBLY FINAL) VISIT. IT HAS TAKEN A TOTAL OF 70
MINUTES TO COMPLETE.

INSTRUCTOR 19

Item 10 contains a notion that often provokes hostility among professionals who describe themselves as 'caring'. That is the notion of 'minimum involvement'. For some reason many professionals believe that they must do all they have time to do for people with problems, though without thinking through their view that this is 'good' professional practice: it tends to be done for its own sake. If we recognise that professionals do not have ownership of problems and that it is the primary managers (parents) who sort out problems, there is nothing to be gained by giving a contrary impression to parents.

The professionals' task is to advise.

If trainees argue that the caring professions need always to be available to help with every problem, it would be an idea to ask them to make a list of five reasons and then submit these to open discussion.

The central criterion is, 'Do these lead to a resolution of family problems?'.

Objective 2

To provide an example of the ten steps in a real life situation

The purpose of Objective 2 is to provide an example of a problem being managed through the ten steps provided in Objective 1.

HANDOUT 16

The Jones family

Mr Jones in his early thirties, is a fitter for the gasboard. Six years younger, Mrs Jones works afternoons in a local newsagent's shop. There are two children, Katie (2 years) and Olwyn (4 years). Mrs Jones' mother looks after the children in the afternoon.

Both parents say Katie is the perfect child. She is charming, quiet, intelligent and pretty. Olwyn is noisy, disobedient, has tantrums when things do not go her own way, and is violent towards Katie.

Evenings in the Jones household are said to be a nightmare. Katie goes to bed quietly and without fuss at 7pm. Mr and Mrs Jones would like Olwyn in bed by 8pm but they have never managed to achieve this and have given up trying because, when they did try, Olwyn flew in a violent temper and then ran away. Now Mr and Mrs Jones believe it is easier not to press and to wait until she falls asleep on the settee before taking her to bed (usually about 11pm).

Even without pressure to go to bed, evenings with Olwyn are very trying. Like most tired children she is touchy, tearful and uncooperative. Tantrums at this time are common when she is thwarted and she hits out at people and objects when they do not bend to her will.

Mr and Mrs Jones try very hard to defuse difficult situations. For example, they try to give Olwyn everything she wants in order to avoid tantrums. They have found this works very well and when they do it tantrums are rare. (Incidentally, Olwyn has about three cups of orange juice each evening: refusing this is a sure way to produce a tantrum). When Olwyn hits out at Mr and Mrs Jones they try to cuddle her and be nice to her. Mr Jones read somewhere that children who hit their parents are looking for love and attention. Mr Jones thinks this must be working because Olwyn seems to like it.

INSTRUCTOR 20

The story in Handout 16 is a typical problem. Although it is only a brief summary, it contains all the relevant information necessary to follow the ten steps—plus a measure of red-herrings.

In the following text pages, each step is taken one at a time and 'what happened' and why is detailed.

Instructors are advised to ask the trainees to determine each step before using 'what happened' as an example. To help the trainees to provide their own answers, instructors should take on the role of parents or anyone else and be prepared to answer any of the trainees' questions. This procedure was used when the trainees were completing exercises on the Smith family.

In completing the ten steps the trainees may come up with different answers from 'what happened'. This is perfectly acceptable provided the answers match the criteria. The answers given are not the only right answers. However, there are wrong answers and these should be pointed out when they appear in the trainees' work. Since there are a variety of right answers it may be an idea for the group to decide collectively on each step with the instructor guiding the process and recording on a blackboard or overhead projector. It would be interesting then to compare with 'what happened'. If the rules are followed you will be surprised at the similarity between the group's work and 'what happened'.

1 Defining the problem behaviours (PBs)

EXERCISE 1   Make a list of the five main problems.

What happened

Arriving at a list of problems proved difficult. This was chiefly because Mr Jones was absorbed with what he had read about 'problem children' being in desperate need of love and attention and at first all he wanted was professional guidance on how to give it more effectively.

After considerable discussion Mr Jones accepted the possibility that Olwyn perhaps did need love and attention but that it was just as likely she needed it because she behaved badly rather than the other way round. The basis of this argument was that Olwyn's behaviour meant she was always in conflict with her parents and seldom getting positive attention. He accepted that it would be better to give her lots of love and attention for behaving well rather than for behaving badly.

The main problems agreed were:

1   Olwyn has a tantrum (hits, screams, hand-bites) when she does not get her own way.

2   Olwyn goes to bed at 11pm each evening.

3   Olwyn hits Katie and makes her cry.

4   Olwyn throws toys around the living room.

5   Olwyn runs away when parents try to put her to bed.

2 Choosing a priority

EXERCISE 2(a)   Which one of the above five would you choose as a priority? Say why. (Your list of five should be pretty much the same apart from how the problems are expressed.)

What happened

The priority was number two: Olwyn goes to bed at 11pm each evening.

All the other problems (except 3) occurred in the evenings when Olwyn should be in bed. If she were in bed, none of them would happen. It is true that the other problems also occurred during the day. But if you stopped say 4 altogether, would this make all that much difference? Moreover, evenings were about the only time parents could relax together. The Jones rarely had this luxury. Were they given this breathing space it would give them a chance to be less edgy about Olwyn. Moreover, if Olwyn went to bed at an earlier time it would obviate the Jones' need to reinforce aspects of her bad behaviour (for example giving in to tantrums and providing positive attention for hitting).

There was very little discussion and no disagreement about choosing this priority. The Jones did ask what they were to do about the other problems. They were advised to carry on as at present with these and focus in the meantime on the priority problem behaviour.

EXERCISE 2(b)   Describe the antecedents and consequences to the PB.

What happened

The antecedents were difficult to express. The difficulty was rationalised by describing the antecedent to the PB as being that Olwyn did not go to bed earlier in the evening. The consequences were much clearer: Olwyn got lots of positive attention.

3 Finding a competing behaviour

EXERCISE 3   Specify a competing behaviour for the Jones' priority PB.

What happened

The CB was defined as: Olwyn goes to bed before 8pm every evening and stays there. The reason for this is self evident.

4 Setting baselines

EXERCISE 4   Devise a simple way of recording the PB and CB. Design a chart the parents can fill in for a period of one week.

What happened

The PB was to be recorded in terms of the time Olwyn went to bed each evening and the CB in terms of the number of times Olwyn was in bed by 8pm. The method of recording involved a chart like this:

Week beginning							
Day	1	2	3	4	5	6	7
Time in bed (PB)							
In bed by 8pm (CB)							

For the PB the parents were asked to enter the time each evening when Olwyn went to bed and stayed there. They were asked not to count time when Olwyn went to bed and later got up. (Why, do you think?)

For the CB parents were asked to enter a tick if the 8pm target was achieved.

The chart was drawn on the spot and left with the parents.

This was the end of the first visit and a date, 10 days away, was arranged for the next visit.

5 Determining rewards (and punishers)

EXERCISE 5   Make up charts (list no more that four items) of rewards and punishers.

If you are doing this without instructors you will have to imagine suitable rewards and punishers. If you are part of a group with instructors then the instructors should take on the roles of the Jones and tell you the sort of things they think Olwyn will work for.

What happened

At first the Jones said that there was nothing Olwyn liked enough to change her behaviour for and that punishment meant absolutely nothing to her. However, discussion revealed that possible rewards were presently available to Olwyn; all her toys, favourite TV programmes, foods and so on were given when she asked for them, irrespective of her behaviour. They agreed to start afresh by making certain favourites available only contingent on good behaviour.

1   A Smartie.

2   Cuddles, hugs, praise from mum and dad.

3   A bedtime story from dad.

4   Taking an old mail order catalogue to bed.

The list you draw up for the exercise might be completely different. This does not matter as long as your rewards are practical, modest and capable of being delivered immediately when Olwyn goes to bed before 8pm.

The punishers were determined on the basis that when Olwyn produced the PB or failed to produce the CB a disincentive must be provided. The list was:

1   No adult attention after 8pm other than putting to bed.

2   All toys, games and other activities put away out of reach at 8pm.

3   No television after 8pm.

4   Confined to living room.

6 Setting up a method of intervention

EXERCISE 6   Summarise in not more than 100 words the key features of an intervention method.

What happened

Olwyn was told exactly what was going on: the behaviour her parents were trying to stop and what they were trying to get her to do instead. The rewards and punishments were explained.

Throughout each day (four or five times) Olwyn was reminded that the target was for her to be in bed before 8pm. For the hour before getting ready she was reminded in ways she would be able to understand in terms of time. For example, you have to get ready 'when this TV programme finishes'.

Before 8pm one of the Jones accompanied Olwyn to wash and change and then get into bed. If Olwyn did not go of her own accord she was taken, undressed and washed and put to bed forcibly.

If Olwyn managed to go to bed without having to be forced then a reward from the menu was given to her. As it turned out, parents found it best to ask Olwyn which one of the four rewards on the menu she preferred on any successful night. Correctly, they made a big production out of giving the reward. Mr and Mrs Jones also chose to use star charting with a star being fixed to a chart above Olwyn's bed on successful nights.

When Olwyn was not in bed by 8pm she was not rewarded and no star was given, even if she was only one minute late. When she had to be forced to bed she was left to cry. On one occasion, Mr Jones had to sit silently outside her door to make sure that Olwyn did not get out.

7 Maintaining the recording system

What happened

For a period of 4 weeks Mr and Mrs Jones recorded the times Olwyn was in bed by 8pm. This was just a continuation of the baseline. In the first week Olwyn was in bed only once by 8pm. In week 4 she was in bed by 8pm every night except one, when she was allowed up for a special event.

8 Go back to baselines

What happened

In week 5, the intervention was stopped and the original baseline condition repeated for one week. In fact, it was not possible to stop the intervention completely since Olwyn had come to look forward very much to a bedtime story from her father, and to getting stars. The repeated baseline showed Olwyn was in bed every night by 8pm.

9 Modifying or maintaining the intervention

What happened

In this case the intervention appeared to be working so no modification was considered.

The main question was whether or not to keep it up. The parents felt that continuing with the full formal intervention (recording, reward menu, reminders during the day, etc) was not necessary. However they said they would continue insisting on an 8pm bedtime and they would keep up the bedtime stories. If things regressed they felt confident they could repeat the process themselves.

10 Discussing progress with parents

What happened

Although the Jones elected not to continue the intervention, their handling of Olwyn had changed considerably. They had learned a new set of problem management techniques which they were beginning to use as a matter of course without seeing them as being a single method of solving a particular problem.

This was discussed with the Jones who resolutely maintained that now that 'the problem' was solved they were going back to normal and apart from the period of intervention they had not changed what they did at all. It did not occur to the Jones that, for example, they were now insisting unswervingly on an 8pm bedtime, and that now Olwyn was being rewarded (the bedtime story) for making it on time.

HANDOUT 17

**Multiple
choice test
on Part 3**

1   The first step in setting up a programme for intervention is:
    (a)   Measure the problem.
    (b)   Define the problem.
    (c)   Find out what is wrong with the child.
    (d)   Set the baseline.

2   A competing behaviour is:
    (a)   A behaviour that needs to be stopped.
    (b)   A sporting activity.
    (c)   Any good behaviour.
    (d)   A behaviour that cannot be done at the same time as the problem
          behaviour.

3   The only problem behaviours that can be measured are:
    (a)   Tantrums.
    (b)   Fussy eating.
    (c)   Hitting others.
    (d)   All of them.

4   If an intervention does not work, you should:
    (a)   End your involvement with the family.
    (b)   Try counselling.
    (c)   Take the child to a doctor because something serious must be
          wrong.
    (d)   Look at ways of changing the intervention programme.

5   If parents reject your considered advice:
    (a)   Try to force them to do the right thing.
    (b)   Alert social services.
    (c)   Leave them alone.
    (d)   Storm off in a huff.

6   Recording of problem behaviour:
    (a)   Should continue throughout the intervention.
    (b)   Is carried out by the professional.
    (c)   Should only be done before and after intervention.
    (d)   Takes place only when the parents remember to do it.

7   A bribe is different from a reward because:
    (a)   Bribes are money, rewards are not.
    (b)   Children like bribes, but they do not like rewards.
    (c)   Bribes are easier to give than rewards.
    (d)   Bribes are given to a child for stopping behaving badly, but
          rewards are given for behaving well.

8 One of the main purposes of an intervention programme is to:
  (a) Teach parents to deal with problem behaviour in general.
  (b) Measure behaviour.
  (c) Let children know they must do as they are told.
  (d) Show people how clever you can be.

9 You should see parents:
  (a) As often as you can manage.
  (b) Only when the problem is due to occur.
  (c) Only as much as is necessary.
  (d) When you are free.

10 Rewards must always be accompanied by:
  (a) Praise.
  (b) Sweets.
  (c) Extra helpings of a favourite pudding.
  (d) Crying.

Summary of Part 3

Ten steps to constructing an intervention were outlined:

1 Defining problem behaviour.

2 Choosing a priority.

3 Finding a competing behaviour.

4 Setting baselines.

5 Determining rewards.

6 Establishing a method of intervention.

7 Maintaining the recording system.

8 Going back to baselines.

9 Modifying and maintaining the intervention.

10 Discussing the outcome.

These were applied in the case of the Jones family. Part 4 goes on to look at the training of parents in skills necessary for successful completion of these steps.

Answers to multiple choice test on Part 3

1 (b)	6 (a)
2 (d)	7 (d)
3 (d)	8 (a)
4 (d)	9 (c)
5 (c)	10 (a)

Trainees should obtain nine points or more before moving on to Goal 4. A score of seven or less suggests the need for a substantial revision of Goal 3.

Further reading on Part 3

S. B. Gordon and W. Davidson, 'Behavioural parent training', in A. S. Gurman and Kristern (eds), *Handbook of Family Therapy* (New York: Brunner–Mazell, 1980).
P. E. Randall and C. Gibb, 'Behaviour Problems, Everybody's Concern', *Health Visitor, Midwife & Community Nurse*, 1988.

PART 4

To provide a method for parent training

This goal is subserved by three objectives:

1 To stress the role of parents in bringing about change.

2 To provide a protocol for transmission of problem management skills to parents.

3 To highlight boobytraps and pitfalls in training parents.

These should be worked through in order before attempting the multiple choice questionnaire on Part 4.

Objective 1

To stress the role of parents in bringing about change

Part 3 was concerned with deriving and constructing a programme of intervention. Part 4 deals with how this, and all it involves, can best be delivered to parents. Objective 1 is aimed at stressing to parents that they are the people who will solve the problem and that no-one else can solve it for them.

Who solves problems

The short answer to this is: the people who have them. In the case of children's behaviour it is the parents who have to face the problems and so ultimately it is the parents who have to solve them.

Unfortunately, with so many professional services available, many parents have the impression that someone else will solve their problems for them. Even more unfortunately many professionals seems to encourage this by taking on 'ownership' of the children's problems in the cases they deal with.

In these circumstances real and lasting resolution of problems becomes impossible. Parents have handed over to an outsider to solve a problem he or she never has to face.

THE PROBLEMS THAT CHILDREN PRESENT BELONG TO THE PARENTS.

The professional's main problem is always: how can I best help and advise these parents as they try to solve their problem?

While the problems faced by parents will vary from child to child and family to family, the professional's problem is always the same.

INSTRUCTOR 21

The preceding text contains a simple message: parents take action to solve behaviour problems; professionals take action to help them do it.

There is a clear distinction here which is not always understood and sometimes even when it is understood it is deliberately ignored by professionals who explicitly claim ownership as a necessary part of practice. Such ownership invariably leads parents further down the road of passivity—a referral made is a responsibility discharged—and the professional into an ever deepening morass of irrelevant detail.

Instructors should try to provoke a discussion on this 'ownership' issue. The main points to bring out concern why a professional should not take on ownership of behaviour problems.

PART 4
OBJECTIVE 1

Establishing 'ownership'

Not all parents who ask for help will be expecting the professional to solve the problem for them. Nevertheless, the ground rules for 'ownership' must be established at the outset of any involvement.

1   The professional should describe his or her job to the parents. Most people outside a particular profession are largely unaware of its basic features. What information they do have is often inaccurate and loaded with unreal expectations.

Basic information includes who employs you, what for and the type of problems on which you can advise. The nature of this will of course vary from profession to profession.

2   The professional should summarise how the present case came his or her way. For example, 'Your GP got in touch with me to say you were having some problems with your daughter, Anne. He tells me you asked for advice because of tantrums and that you agreed to him asking me to call on you ...'.

This summary is very important. It is not unusual for parents to be unaware of how you come to be there. Often other professionals have assumed the parents would like to see you without actually establishing whether or not they would! Moreover, problems can be like Chinese whispers: the parents may be quite surprised at what you have been told about them and their problems. An atmosphere of openness must be established.

3   Having outlined a general role, the professional should outline his or her role in this particular case. This is the first opportunity to express explicitly an advisory, demonstration-type role.

4   The professional should establish that the parents understand and accept the role. It should not be automatically assumed that they will. Many people equate all professional practice with medical practice where, to a greater or lesser extent, a professional does do the solving. If parents do not accept your role there is little you can do.

Objective 2

To provide a protocol for transmission of problem management skills to parents

What follows is a set of steps for introducing parents to running a programme designed to correct problem behaviour(s). The most perfectly designed and constructed intervention programme is valueless unless the parents accept it.

HANDOUT 19

Nine steps *The groundwork*

These steps start after:

(a) Objective 1 of Part 4 has been completed and it is clear who 'owns' the problem.

(b) The first six steps of Part 3, Objective 1, have been completed, up to the point where an intervention programme has been written.

The steps

1 Write the programme in a simple, brief and straightforward manner. (This may be done on the spot or brought at a second visit.)

2 Go through the programme point by point with the parents to make sure:

(a) You are not asking the impossible.

(b) Everyone understands what is to be done.

3 The central idea to transmit is that any programme is a formal device through which rewards can be provided when the problem does not occur in circumstances where sometimes it does, and through which disincentives are provided whenever the problem does occur.

4 Stress consistency in delivering these rewards and disincentives. This is closely related to how realistic the programme is. The parents must agree that they can deliver the rewards and disincentives always and not just sometimes.

5 Always try to give a practical demonstration of how to use the programme. For example, suppose the programme focuses on a child who does not obey saying that he will learn to do so after one telling. It is recommended the professional demonstrate 'how' to the parents. In this case it may be by asking the child to pick up a toy, being ignored, then compelling him or her to pick it up by physical guidance then putting the child out of the room and leaving him when the inevitable tantrum occurs.

Parents are encouraged by seeing a perceived expert being as firm as they would like to be and not being put off by the resulting tantrum.

6 Emphasise the importance of continued record keeping. The details of this should not present problems since the parents will have kept a baseline already.

7 Arrange to visit after the programme has had a few weeks to run.

8 Re-visit and consider modifying or maintaining the programme.

9 Reinforce the parents. This is vitally important. You will be asking them to do something difficult and unusual for them. Their efforts should be appreciated.

INSTRUCTOR   22

These steps can be role played as a prompter for group discussion.

It is important to stress to the trainees that the steps are not separate from the process described in Part 3. The whole thing is interlinked.

Objective 3

To highlight boobytraps and pitfalls in parents' training

There are many things that can go wrong when training parents, or anybody else for that matter. This section aims to highlight some of these things.

INSTRUCTOR 23

Some typical errors and boobytraps are given on the following pages. However, these are by no means the only pitfalls a professional is likely to encounter. There will be others, especially related to particular families.

It is impossible to explore all the possible pitfalls. The instructor is advised to encourage the trainees to generate others and to submit them to group discussion.

The following text pages can be used by the instructor as prompts to the discussion.

Potential pitfalls and boobytraps

OWNERSHIP
It is only necessary now simply to reiterate this pitfall and say the professional must be aware of it from the outset of contact with parents.

THE GO-BETWEEN
It is not unusual for parents to find professionals wanting. Perhaps this is because they really are wanting or perhaps it is because the professional refuses to take on a role that the parents want but that he or she thinks unsuitable. The professional here is in danger of becoming a go-between in that parents may say, 'If you can't help perhaps you will refer us to someone who can!' If parents want this they can do it themselves. They will, if they try hard enough, always find someone to do their bidding.

Of course, there will be times when, having considered a problem, you think it is outside your remit. In these cases referring on is suitable. The difference is that here you have made a professional decision.

COERCION
Sometimes when a professional gives considered advice parents exercise their right to reject it. Parents are within their rights to make such a

decision: apart from anything else it is their child and they own the problem. Their choice should be respected.

Professionals who try to coerce parents into acting on advice they have rejected should ask themselves what they hope to achieve.

If parents reject advice—and assuming you cannot compromise your professional judgement—respect them and leave.

OVER-SUPPORT All of us like to receive support from others when we have a problem, even if it is only talking things over with friends. Parents need this support too. But the support is not being available whenever parents ask for help. Being too available can be counterproductive. What the professional is doing is offering a framework within which parents can learn skills to solve their own problems. The support given should be that necessary to carry out your objectives. In fact, support may consist of saying 'I leave you to work out an answer to that problem'.

COMPLEXITY Human functioning is very complex and little is known about it. This does not mean that action to solve human problems has to be equally complex. In fact, since so little is known about human functioning there is no point in being complex about problem-solving. The more complex professional action becomes, the less likely it is to have any effect. Strive for simplicity: parents may well be impressed by 'mystique' to start with but it will soon become a joke when it fails to produce the goods.

RELIABILITY If people who promise to telephone or visit you fail to do so it is very annoying. Such failure must be especially annoying to parents who are worried about their child. How often have you heard parents say, 'Nobody took us seriously when we told them about the problem?' If you make an arrangement, keep it.

114

HANDOUT 20

Multiple choice test on Part 4

1 The person who solves problems is:
   (a) Usually the GP.
   (b) The parents.
   (c) The professional.
   (d) The child.

2 It is a good idea for a professional to:
   (a) Deal with children as if they were his or her own.
   (b) Be firm with parents whose home is untidy.
   (c) Explore parents' feelings about their problem.
   (d) Assist parents in dealing with their problem.

3 The problem the professional faces is:
   (a) That the child's family is on supplementary benefit.
   (b) To stop children's bad behaviour.
   (c) How best to help and advise parents as they try to solve their problem.
   (d) That so many people are poor and so cannot be expected to manage behaviour problems

4 The first time a professional meets parents he or she should:
   (a) Say what his or her job is and what he or she does.
   (b) Not waste time and get straight at the problem.
   (c) Inspect the home for signs of mismanagement.
   (d) Arrive with a colleague.

5 The key components of the professional's role are:
   (a) To be expert, decisive, masterful and firm.
   (b) To offer advice, guidance, a management framework and demonstrations.
   (c) To be flexible and ever-responsive to parents' wishes.
   (d) Steadfastness, integrity, subtlety and guile.

6 Parents are:
   (a) Always ready to accept what professionals say.
   (b) To blame for badly behaved children.
   (c) Grown people who are capable of thinking for themselves and making their own decisions.
   (d) Usually in need of emotional support.

7 Practical demonstrations of dealing with problem behaviour:
   (a) Are always a good idea.
   (b) Show children who is boss.
   (c) Usually solve the problem.
   (d) Help parents to do it themselves.

8 Parents should be congratulated for managing their problem:
   (a) Because praise is one of the things that will help them keep it up.
   (b) Because they like it.
   (c) Even if they did not do anything.
   (d) When you feel in a good mood.

9 Professionals should resist becoming 'go-betweens' because:
   (a) They do not have the time.
   (b) Parents are capable of doing it themselves.
   (c) It is too difficult.
   (d) Research evidence shows that people who become go-betweens
        cannot tell the difference between margarine and butter.

10 Solutions to problems should always be:
    (a) Complex.
    (b) Simple.
    (c) Capable of being carried out.
    (d) Shrouded in professional mystique.

Summary of Part 4

Essentially, Part 4 was about negotiating with parents. The first aspect covered was to do with who owns problems and the notion that it is parents, not professionals. Second, nine steps to use as a guide when introducing parents to an intervention were detailed. Third, a range of sample pitfalls and boobytraps was described. The idea here was that forewarned is forearmed and that problems are less likely to occur if clear practice is used from the outset.

Answers to multiple choice test on Part 4

1 (b)	6 (c)
2 (d)	7 (d)
3 (c)	8 (a)
4 (a)	9 (b)
5 (b)	10 (c)

Trainees should score nine or more. A score of seven or less suggests revision is necessary.

Further reading on Part 4

M. Herbert, *Behavioural Treatment of Children with Problems: A Practice Manual* (London: Academic Press, 1987).
P. E. Randall, 'In Charge', *Community Care* (1987).
K. Hewitt and W. Crawford, 'Resolving Behaviour Problems in Pre-School Children: Evaluation of a Workshop for Health Visitors,' *Child Care, Health & Development*, **14**, (1988) 1–10.

PART 5

> ## Test your strength

The final part provides a description of a family problem through which to try out what has been learned in the preceding parts.

The story of the Smith family, first introduced in Part 1, is presented again and you are asked to write a protocol that follows the ten steps in Part 3 and makes use of the information in Parts 1, 2 and 4.

INSTRUCTOR 24

Handout 21 contains a description of the Smith family and some of their problems. It is the same as Handout 1 apart from the accompanying questions and instructions.

Instructors should distribute Handout 21 and ask trainees to write a protocol for a possible intervention using what they have learned in the preceding parts—particularly the ten steps in Part 3.

Trainees should have at least a week to complete this but they can be helped with a list of the key components their responses should contain:

1 The sequence of steps given in Part 3.

2 Clear identification of a priority problem behaviour (PB) and a competing behaviour (CB).

3 A recording system that is objective, uncomplicated and replicable.

4 Suggestions of suitable reward (a 'menu').

5 An intervention which attempts to replace the PB with the CB.

6 A means of maintaining the recording system during the intervention.

It is advisable that the date set for completion involves a group meeting and discussion of possible responses. This may be guided by the subsequent text pages which describe the intervention that was carried out by the Smiths. It should be stressed that this is not the only possible intervention. What is important is that the trainees follow the same principles.

HANDOUT 21

The Smith family

Write a protocol for possible intervention with the Smiths using the information in the preceding four parts, particularly the ten steps in Part 3.

1   The family consists of:

Mr George Smith, 36 years old, unemployed for 2½ years.

Mrs Susan Smith, 25 years old, housewife.

Amy Smith, 11 months old.

Keith Smith, 4 years old.

Andrew Smith, 15 years old, currently in the closed unit of a community home with education.

2   Mr Smith has been married twice and Andrew is his son by his first marriage. It ended in a stormy divorce after three years when the first Mrs Smith walked out leaving the then 4-year-old Andrew locked in a wardrobe. She has had no real contact since but occasionally rings up Mr Smith and Andrew to enquire how her 'bairn' is getting on. She sounds intoxicated and frequently weeps. These telephone calls provoke long and furious rows between Mr Smith and his second wife.

Mr Smith is unemployed. He says he was made redundant from his storeman job but Mrs Smith says he was sacked for being drunk. He seems to spend most of his day doing little other than occasionally walking to the pub (usually in the middle of a row) where he can spend up to 3 hours. He has had only sporadic, unskilled labouring work since leaving school but he did have, for 18 months, a job as a taxi driver with a friend. He claims this was the best time of his life.

He seems to be a bit strange and possibly mildly depressed.

Mr Smith complains that his second wife is lazy. He is annoyed that she does little cleaning and that the burden of getting Keith and Amy up and breakfasted is always his responsibility. He then takes Keith to his morning nursery class.

Mr Smith complains that Mrs Smith is frigid. They have little or no sexual contact and only rarely do they express their feelings for each other.

He is begging for help. His financial state is bad and poor management has led to lump sum payments from the DHSS to cover electricity and other bills. He is terrified that Keith is 'going the same way as Andrew' and feels frustrated and emasculated, because he cannot control either of his sons' behaviour.

3   Mrs Susan Smith is considerably younger. She had had many boyfriends before meeting Mr Smith and lived with him for about one year before they married, five months before Keith was born.

Mrs Smith is attractive in a jaded way and exudes a cheerful demeanour that is out of proportion to the magnitude of her problems. She complains bitterly about Mr Smith saying that he is 'a lazy, good-for-nothing drunk' whose first wife 'had the best years of him'. She feels that he does not appreciate her and that he should be grateful to have a good looking young wife. At present she is very worried about her stretch marks which have not faded since Amy's birth. These embarrass her when she changes at her adult education course of aerobics. She is also concerned that Amy is not putting on weight and that Keith disregards her. She has stopped Keith from having cold drinking chocolate which he adores because a neighbour said that the additives might be making him hyperactive. She would like to talk to her own mother about the children, but there is no contact at the moment because Mr Smith told Susan's mother to '.... off' when he thought she was interfering in the family.

Susan is on the pill but wonders why she bothers when her husband is so sexually inactive.

4   Keith is a good looking but scruffy 4-year-old who goes to a nursery unit (attached to a primary school) five mornings a week. The staff there say that he is hyperactive and aggressive. They believe that his hostility is caused by frustration; apparently he will not play very long at any activity and his speech is unclear.

At home Keith is a naughty boy and frequently has breath holding tantrums to which his parents have responded by smacking and shouting at him. On one occasion they locked him in a bedroom and he threw a wooden brick through a window and tore down the curtains. He is clearly a very disturbed and emotionally rejected child because he deliberately urinates on the carpets and bedding, refuses to go to bed or stay in his own bed. His tempers at nighttime disturb Amy and also earn bangs on the wall from the irritated but otherwise kindly, elderly couple next door. Keith will play with Amy but woe betide her if she does not hand him toys, her food etc.

Keith has his good side—he laughs a lot and plays in a limited way with a toy garage, cars and some Lego. He is always pleased to see his nursery teacher but is terrified that she will think he is a naughty boy. He likes watching TV with his father and is keen to talk to the latter about the programmes they see together.

5   Amy is a delightful child and is the reason for frequent visits from the health visitor. She cries a lot and is not putting on weight. Her play seems to lack imagination and she is manifestly terrified of Keith. He seems to intimidate her and he prefers to eat her food and play with her toys.

Her appearance is as ill-kempt as the rest of the home.

6   Andrew, after prolonged and rather unintelligent delinquency, has been placed in the secure unit of a community house with education. He absconds frequently, returning home to display acting-out tendencies. On occasions he seems wistful and quiet but his attitude is definitely and generally antisocial.

Intervening with the Smith family

The intervention is laid out in terms of the ten steps given in Part 3.

1 SPECIFICATION OF PROBLEM BEHAVIOUR

The marriage is failing with both parties complaining about the lack of affection and sexual contact between them. The ex-wife is ringing up over a son in whom she has shown no interest. Mr Smith feels unable to do anything and Mrs Smith worries about her stretch marks while her world crumbles about her. Both are worried that Keith is embarking on the long downhill road to delinquency and even the nursery staff have resorted to clichés to describe his behaviour.

In initial discussion Mr and Mrs Smith expressed their main problem in broad terms as being that they did not seem to get on well: they were always 'at each other's throats'. Explaining this they went on to say that perhaps if they did not have to put up with Keith's trying behaviour every day until evening they might have fewer rows. Thus:

2 PRIORITY PROBLEM BEHAVIOUR

Keith stays up late at night.

3 COMPETING BEHAVIOUR

Keith goes to bed at 7.30pm each evening and stays there till 7am.

4 SETTING A BASELINE

To do this, the Smiths noted, over one week, the time Keith went to bed (PB) and whether he stayed in bed till 7am.

WEEK 1		Sun	Mon	Tues	Wed	Thur	Fri	Sat
Problem behaviour	Time in bed	11.15	1.30	10.35	10.45	11.00	11.15	11.45
Competing behaviour	Stays in bed until 7am	X	X	X	X	X	X	X

This shows clearly that the problem behaviour is excessive for a child of Keith's age. The crosses in the competing behaviour boxes show that during the baseline week he never stayed in his bed until 7am.

| 5 DETERMINING REWARDS | These were, of course, arrived at in discussion with the Smiths. |

(a) Praise and attention from Mr Smith.
(b) Cold chocolate drinks.
(c) Praise from Keith's nursery teacher for being 'good' at home. It also emerged that Keith hated his nursery teacher to know he had been naughty and that he did not like any form of physical restraint.

| 6 A METHOD OF INTERVENTION | *Week 1 (after the baseline week)* |

(a) Keith was told that if he went up to bed at 9pm his father would read him a story while he had a quarter cup of cold drinking chocolate.
(b) If Keith got out of bed one or other parent would immediately return him and hold him gently but firmly until he lay quietly. This was repeated throughout the night until 7am the next day.

When he had remained in his bed to at least 6.30am he was praised and given a big mug of chocolate.

Subsequent weeks

At the start of week 2 the required time to go to bed was reduced by half an hour and Keith was rewarded only if this new time was achived. This was further reduced in subsequent weeks until the target time of 7.30pm was reached.

The same progressive approach was applied to keep Keith in bed until 7am.

| 7 MAINTAINING THE RECORDING SYSTEM | The same chart was used over a period of 4 weeks. |

| 8 BACK TO THE BASELINE | In the fifth week the original baseline condition (no intervention) was applied for two nights only because it was clear that this problem had virtually disappeared. |

| 9 MODIFYING THE INTERVENTION | This was not necessary. |

| 10 DISCUSSING THE OUTCOME WITH PARENTS | A new priority was chosen and another priority identified. This time the Smiths took a greater part in designing an intervention and deciding what they were to do. |

SUMMING UP

If there is a single most important component of this course it is the notion that parents, not professionals, solve problems.

The professional's role is not to be the 'expert' who comes in to put things right. The aim of any professional involvement must always be to advise and assist parents in solving their own problems.

Helping parents in this way is an attempt to provide them with child-management skills for life so that they can generate solutions to many of the problems they face without reference to professionals at all. In the tenth step of the Smith family intervention, the Smiths were beginning to generalise the skills they had learned in the process of getting Keith to bed and persuading him to stay there. Even if an intervention is successful in solving a discrete problem like this, the whole process cannot be counted as a success if every step has to be repeated for the next discrete problem.

Whatever the nature of the immediate problem, the professional must always have an eye to helping parents generalise the skills they have learned.

That has been the focus of this course and we hope we have managed to provide a framework for practice within which this can be achieved.

Index